CLEMENS KUBY

Healthy without medicine

CLEMENS KUBY

Healthy without medicine

The KUBYmethod – a manual for thinking differently

Note: The information, recommendations, and practice suggestions contained in this book are intended to increase consciousness. However, they cannot replace a medical diagnosis and appropriate treatment for which a qualified specialist must be consulted if necessary. The author and publisher point out that self-treatment is your own responsibility. Liability for damage of any kind arising from ignoring this information is hereby excluded.

Healthy without medicine

Translation: Margit Loerzer
Proofreading: Liz Marino
Author Photo: Astrid Kuby
Illustrations: Herbert Beier
Typesetting: Kai Rübsamen
Printing: Amazon.com, Inc. Kindle direct publishing

ISBN Paperback: 978-3-932486-32-6
ISBN mobi: 978-3-932486-31-9
ISBN epub: 978-3-932486-33-3

www.clemenskuby.com

If you want to change something, you have to look to yourself first.

Contents

Foreword 8

As I think, I am 13

Mind and matter 14

"What would people think?" 18

Information for all cells 25

Five human images 30

"Better not talk about it ..." 34

Choosing to be healthy 41

The soul wants truthfulness and not profiteering 42

Intuition – the royal road to knowledge 49

"I've got it under control." 50

Recognising and using your own competence 57

"But somebody has to do it!" 61

The KUBYmethod 69

Soul writing 70

Two self-healing stories 89

A script for the new reality 101

Self-love is the beginning of all love 105

Compassion begins with feeling 106

Everything is fine just as it is 112

"We do not show weakness." 115

"Can I allow myself that?" 121

Appendix 129

How does Soul Writing work exactly? 130

About the author 137

Contact 139

Foreword

Dear Reader,

"Healthy without Medicine!" Is that even possible? Why do the pharmaceutical industry and the comprehensive medical network even exist if we could all heal without them? Healing without conventional medical treatments and without medicines of any kind whatsoever, without any material input – is that even possible?

If we had been told about 30 years ago that phones would work without British Telecom or AT&T and without a nationwide network, we would certainly have also been very sceptical. Hardly anyone could imagine that without a stationary device and without a telephone booth, everyone can communicate with a small, cordless box anytime, anywhere. Many would have thought it absolutely unreal to see the other side of the globe live in picture and sound with such a mobile device even a few years ago. And today? Smartphones are a given.

There is a right time for everything. And each age has its own level of consciousness. But consciousness does not develop straightforwardly, but in leaps and bounds. Our collective leap into the age of communication was achieved with the Internet. Our leap into the spiritual age will be achieved with self-healing without medicine. With spiritual consciousness, matter (the body) is subordinated to the mind, and thus we have the omnipotence of the spirit. This jump in consciousness should not be a cause for fear or aggression, but a source of joy. We welcome the change, because in it lies the meaning of our life and it is the only thing that remains.

Unfortunately, many people are not aware of the change in consciousness until their former concepts are no longer working – which leads to unnecessary pain. It was no different for me: in 1981, I was paralysed after a serious accident. The prognosis was "wheelchair for life". Despite the best care, only when there was no more hope that I would ever walk again did my consciousness change, and the medicine free *KUBY™method*, as you will find in this book in short form, came into existence. This leap of consciousness was forced upon me in a way. On the one hand, because I could walk again without surgery and without any medication, and on the other hand because I had made films since I was 21.

In cinema, there is also no material intervention, and yet the body reacts. Many people really cry in the cinema. For some, their pulse and heart begin to race even though they are sitting comfortably in a chair, but their spirits are thinking: "Someone's about to die." Everyone knows that it's just pretend, but the physical reaction is real. I was even told of a case where after one of my films a woman "forgot" her crutches in the cinema and has since been able to walk normally, something no one had previously thought possible.

I have produced more than 50 consciousness expanding films and have taught film for 5 years at university. I had to learn that reality does not need to be "real", rather reality is what has an effect. Our brain cannot distinguish between fact and fiction, and there is a divine or inconceivably great potential to heal ourselves in a purely spiritual way. In the many years of my seminar practice, there have been countless people who have healed with the *KUBYmethod*, purely mentally, even from the most serious diseases.

No physical means are needed for it, no operations, not even hands are laid upon you; no two points on the body have to be touched, and no religious concepts have to be followed. The *KUBYmethod* changes the human image. If you've believed until now that people are bio-chemical beings, then that is also how you will be treated. But with the *KUBYmethod* humans are recognised as spiritual beings, and then medicine no longer plays a part; you fundamentally no longer think materialistically. This is at least as great a step forward in consciousness as going from analogue to digital. Those who don't take this step do not understand smartphones and still hang onto their old analogue fax and telephone. As with the smartphones the *KUBYmethod* opens up a completely different world.

I imagine that you also have the desire to be or become healthy without medicine or at least to learn about it. The instructions for that are already in your hands. For the first time I am specifically taking up female and male perspectives, because practice shows that women and men approach the leap of consciousness in different ways.

Anyone can start experimenting with this book right away. It is best to proceed practically: take a topic that you would like to have clarified now. This is not only true for physical problems; with the *KUBYmethod* it is also possible to solve serious relationship, work, or money problems – something that has been very stressful and/or painful for a long time or at the moment. Make this problem your “project” and take it as a challenge to your personal development.

Thus you can turn a disadvantage into an advantage. For example I saw my accident as the greatest catastrophe of my life. Now it is my greatest treasure. With the *KUBYmethod* you can also do this with your project. Take it step by step. Think about how much time, money, and energy you have spent on fighting symptoms so far. If you use even a fraction of your effort on causative self-healing, you will reach a higher level of being, on which you perceive your self-responsibility through self-competence. In addition, you will find that you can keep refining the *KUBYmethod* throughout your whole life.

I wish you luck and success in this endeavour.

Regards, *Clemens Kuby*
Autumn 2016

1

As I think, I am

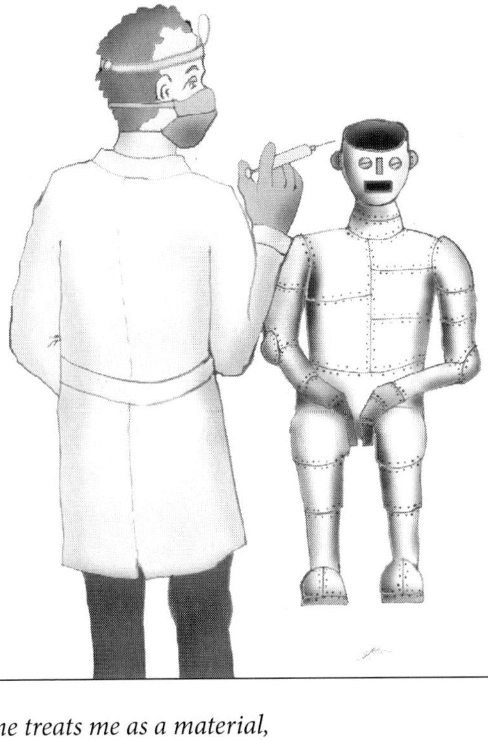

"Medicine treats me as a material, biochemical being."

Mind and matter

If we imagine health without medicine and want to live it and experience it too, we cannot ignore two aspects that are of great importance for physical and mental well-being: mind and matter.

If you recognise matter as the crucial expression and regulator of our existence, you will also rely on the effect of an allopathic or homeopathic drug, a syringe, an operating room, that is, physical input to repair what is no longer working. If spiritual impulses are the main engines of life, you will be looking for other ways because you know or have already learnt that the body is only healthy in the long term if the soul is so as well. "Well fine," you might say, "you can follow both concepts." In practice often, you may agree, but which of the two concepts takes priority? Mind or matter: Which one is the primary force here? Many believe that matter is the authority and it dictates over our living conditions. That this is a mistake becomes clear when we ask ourselves, according to the law of cause and effect: Is mind the cause of matter or matter the cause of mind? Most people are of the opinion that matter does not need a cause; it simply consists of itself. Of course, that cannot be the case in this universe, but this view is widespread. It forms the core of materialism, which medicine is also a part of, and thus also shapes our usual concept of healing.

What does it refer to? This view arises from a matter which, so to speak, has emerged from itself, just as we should believe it happened with the story of the Big Bang theory. This, however, would mean that the chair on which I am sitting, or the bed on which I lie, created itself without cause. This is not possible. Not even imaginable. Anyone who thinks this is possible must believe that a bed or a chair has fallen out of the sky. Just like that – whoops, there's a chair. I think you'll agree with me that there would never be a chair if someone had not had the idea of a chair. Without the idea of a chair, there would never have been a chair in this universe. It is the same with the bed, the tree, the house, the earth, the solar system, and so on.

For everything, a spiritual impulse or an idea was necessary for its development, before materialisation became possible. Without a spiritual impulse, nothing is created, not even the smallest or the greatest things. The Bible says: In the beginning was the Word. It does not say: In the beginning was Matter. Nor does any ancient philosophy or any other religion say this. The Hindu teachings of the Bhagavad Gita, the Buddhist sutras as well as the Koran all say the same as the Bible: **In the beginning is spirit.**

This hierarchy of being can also be deduced quite soberly from the chronology of the phenomenon: if we recognise that matter is always bound to space and time, and spirit / mind is not, then we can ask ourselves: What came first? Space and time or spirit / mind? Space and time are always a finite entity, mind is not. The mind has no beginning or end. So, for this very simple reason, the mind must have been present in space and time in this universe, not just evolutionarily, but also at every moment. These philosophical considerations of principle are also important for understanding how we can change matter, that is, the body, in a spiritual way. The *KUBYmethod* states: self-healing begins with thinking. From what explanation model can the hierarchy of mind and matter be deduced? The mind, as I use this term, means far more than brain activity. The mind is in every atom. We can apply this atomic model to the entire universe. A meteorite that comes from another galaxy and falls to Earth, or material from the Moon or from Mars – we can apply the same atomic structure to everything with its elementary particles and the vacuum as we do on Earth.

Physics has now produced the manifold proof that vacuum is not a vacuum, that is, it is not empty, hollow, and therefore negligible, but possesses a natural oscillation. We can, therefore, assume that something is happening in every atom. How does physics prove spiritual activity? By measuring brain currents (frequencies). It does not know the content of spiritual activity, but it knows that spiritual activity exists.

If we interpret the natural oscillation of an atom in the same way, then every atom is mentally active and not empty, hollow, and virtually dead.

That is why we can also call mind the Great Spirit, because it is in every atom. Spirit as a synonym for the intelligence of the universe. Many call it God. For others it is chi, and for others it is Allah or Buddha. **This spirit is omnipresent and all embracing**. A picture of it would be the ocean which we are in the midst of. The soul is then a cup of water from the ocean, the individualised spirit so to speak: the cup symbolises the body as the vessel for the soul or as its materialised expression. The water in the cup is ocean water and remains ocean water. That is, the soul is also the Great Spirit and the Great Spirit is the soul. What do we learn from this? If I always assume that all beings are spiritual beings, then everything also occurs on the spiritual level: just as I think, I am – that is how the world is, and so is my counterpart, and so is everything.

Mind is therefore always without a beginning and without an end. Only the form has a beginning and thus also an end. But despite this connection between the spiritual cause and the material effect, our attention is mostly directed to the form, including in medicine. We like to stick to the form, that is, to matter, because we can understand it more quickly. We live in a very materialistic time. Only what we can see, weigh, measure, and calculate counts. "Real" is the form or mechanical, biochemical phenomenon. Everything else is rejected as speculation. From the perspective of the mind this is logical and understandable.

Luckily, however, our brains have not only a left hemisphere, with which we are able to think and create rationally, but also a right one. Even if we don't train it, it is still there. With the capabilities of the right hemisphere, we have possibilities without the limitations of space and time. And this is our greatest opportunity to master new challenges. After all, we all want to be or become healthy. There is nothing more important.

If we place priority on our mind, then our thoughts determine how we are and what will become of us. Our own thoughts can be formed much, much more easily than circumstances. The possibilities of shaping life with the mind as the guiding force are therefore so much greater and more diverse that we really ought to want to use this faculty. It is strange that we separate mind from matter and think that matter is something without spirit. This is the same nonsense as defining spirit as "nothing."

WOMEN ONLY

"What would people think?"

Adapting to what others want, self-denial

The woman of today is an independent, emotionally-oriented being who, in a very impressive way, manages the most complex processes in her family and career. Often enough, she mobilises an energy that some men can only dream of. But how does it happen that in particularly delicate situations – for example in the case of serious living decisions or serious health problems – this self-understanding crumbles down in many women and is undermined by doubt?

Whether we like it or not, some women, although settled in life, have a problem with taking their destiny into their own hands. Exceptions, of course, always prove the rule, but I experience in my seminars and elsewhere that strong women react to real independence with great fear: "What will become of me?" "I can't just do this or that?" "What will my husband say about it?" "What will my children think of me?" "But the doctor said that …" "When my mother hears this …" and so on.

Women have learnt to ask – and not to decide for themselves. When their area of expertise is assigned to them, they can accomplish great things. On the other hand, entering new territory on their own is contrary to prevailing female upbringing. There always has been an authority which ultimately decided what was or wasn't allowed. In most cases, the authority did not even have to say it. Daughters, for example, can read from their fathers' expressions (and also their all-determining mothers) what is permissible and what is not, and then, as a matter of course, align themselves accordingly. A lot happens before a woman says: "Now I'm going to do what I want". But does it have to get to the extreme before their self-competence breaks through?

If a woman pushes the adjustment too far and becomes potentially seriously ill, this is first a price too high for independence, and second often so late that it is associated with great sacrifices. If independence is not practised at an early stage, then it is very difficult to apply even in medicine when illness happens. Whether it's a female or male doctor, whitecoats have an authority that women are often willing to give themselves to without contradiction, because they have mainly learnt to define themselves via their bodies. The fact that her own mind (her personal thinking) rules over her body is not taught by fashion nor by her mother, and certainly not by the entire wellness and health programmes found in women's magazines.

A woman is taught to look after her body as best as possible. When the doctor says what her supposedly sick body needs or does not need, a woman socialised in this way quickly loses her self-confidence. In a situation where she is in pain, it is very hard for her to say, "I am my own boss, especially when it comes to my body." This would require a completely different way of thinking. Instead, the responsibility is rather – as learnt – deferred to the view that the medical doctor ultimately possesses the highest and, above all, ultimate competence in matters regarding the body.

Perhaps you may be wondering how this can change? First and foremost, by making a so-called egoistical decision in the very best sense: namely, by putting yourself first. Women always flinch if they are called "egoistical". They do not like it because they prefer to fit into the typical image of the all-round lady/maternal figure. New ideas are not well-received – and if they are, only when others agree. Approval granted – when a woman feels it´s safe to proceed.

Healthy egoism, however, looks different. It consists of paying attention to your own soul's needs, the one that has no existential angst and no *"what will people think?"*-fears. Recognising these needs provides the competency for your own well-being, which puts every outside opinion into perspective.

Such a development starts with getting out of your usual energy field, otherwise, other thoughts and feelings will be superimposed on the voice of your soul, and you would not find out what is trying to tell you. To be able to hear your soul, you can use your high body awareness as follows: stop focusing on the outside, but concentrate on finding your inner self – very soon you will then realise what is right for you and what is wrong for you. After this takes place, you only need the courage to implement such a realisation.

And you will have this courage as soon as you have moved out of the usual energy field. *Soulwriting* will certainly be able to help you here. Do not wait until the water is up to your neck for you to take your destiny into your own hands with the courage that only comes from despair. You can and may make it easier for yourself.

To free yourself from too much adjustment and to act on your own does not mean ignoring all other opinions. With more self-confidence, new points of view can be recognised and integrated into your own decisions – including and especially on health issues: when you are ill, always be aware of what kind of advice you seek. A physical diagnosis of the symptom or guidance to help yourself? Treatment for the symptoms or healing the root cause? Different people are responsible for each area. You cannot complain that no pears grow on an apple tree. A doctor tells you only what they have learnt, never what your soul has to say (doctors are not trained for this – exceptions prove the rule). This means: YOU decide from which source you want advice, and then look for the relevant people to discuss it with. This is already the first step towards self-competence.

Whatever happens, you say, "I've made it this far, I can go further. I know that I must be even more consistent in my self-responsible life in order to be completely healed. The soul – my soul – wants full happiness, and that is what I will now allow myself. "Do you want this? Well, then make the decision and take your destiny into your own hands!

After many 4years of practice with the *KUBYmethod* and countless seminars in which people always show surprising successes with self-healing, I can summarise: *consciousness changes matter*. This puts me in agreement with modern physics. This is calming and contributes to not doubting or even despairing over the experience.

Let us, therefore, take the opportunity to take care of our health right away! I consider prevention to be the most effective way to provide modest resources for a much healthier society. This begins with children. If we do not let their right brain hemisphere waste away, they can gain controlled, intuitive experiences that give them a lifelong human image with which they can shape a happy and healthy life.

But as adults we can still learn how to create our own responsibility, our own reality, thoughtfully and intuitively. The function of our proportionally oversized brain, which consumes 20% of our energy but only 3% of our mass, is what creates our reality. Research has found that more than 90% of our perception comes from our own experience treasure, which consists of our beliefs, prejudices, impressions, and expectations. The primary function of our five sense organs is therefore not to perceive reality, but to confirm our prejudices. So let's take advantage of that. If we steer our perception from our spiritual experience, we clear up our store of knowledge so that it is a positive perception of our reality. And not just illness, but also health and happiness are part of our reality.

The problem for materialists is that they believe in an objective reality that exists independently of their perception. Such people therefore only have a very small scope for change. For example they cannot retroactively change what happened before. They seek an external influence for each change. And even that offers them only a few possibilities for change, because they are dependent on a bio-chemical, materialistic input, which has an effect on their bio-chemical, materialistic being. They are fundamentally lacking the conviction that they can also achieve material, physical, and bio-chemical effects through spiritual input.

But these people would be able to reject this conviction completely the next time they see a movie, because they have probably already cried during a movie or sat next to someone who did. And perhaps they were wondering why real tears were being shed, when what triggered the tears was, of course, an illusion. Every thinking person knows that none of the actors die in reality. And yet, as I mentioned in my foreword, they believe in the illusion so much that, in addition to tears, symptoms such as a racing heart, sweating, etc. also occur. This means that even **the greatest materialist is a spiritual being** and their physical responses are controlled by purely spiritual input. This is what people are paying for when they buy their movie ticket. And they prefer the films in which the projected illusion produces the strongest reactions in them.

I have been a filmmaker for over 40 years and I know what I'm talking about, because I've studied this mechanism in depth. This also included the fact that for 23 years, I have been researching all over the world how spontaneous healing, that is healing through mental cures is even possible. I have documented a total of 360 hours of mental healing processes, which resulted in my cinema documentary *En route to the next dimension* and later also the book of the same name.

But even after the film, I was still not fully aware of how in my own and other cases spiritual healing actually works. Another film with modern brain researchers and Buddhist teachers was necessary. Through them, I finally understood what shamans, healers, magicians, and medicine men and women all over the world do. They do exactly what our brain research has always shown: **we do not have our great brain to perceive reality, but to create it**. Such a creative process is commonly referred to as "illusion." However, since this term has a negative association, I prefer to use the word *imagination*. And so I say today, after all my experiences: if real physical reactions can be evoked through imagination, then we should also use this ability to heal ourselves physically! Materialists, therefore, by no means have to renounce their much-lauded science and rationality. Because it is only too understandable that they are always looking for something solid, objective, and measurable because they have forgotten their intuition due to the extreme interpretation of European Enlightenment. It is not about rejecting matter and reason, it is about subordinating it to the mind (to which intuition and the soul belong).

Visions and ideas always come from intuition, as already mentioned. **We need reason so that ideas and visions can be converted into matter.** Without reason, we can do nothing, but the mind is in charge – as it is for our physical health and other health related matters. Existence is not what determines consciousness, but consciousness existence. It is therefore crucial not to proclaim an either-or, but merely to acknowledge that our brain has two very effective halves – the rational on the left, intuition on the right. *Both* want to be activated to achieve the best results – in all areas of life. Let us use this potential!

Information for all cells

There are infinite examples of the brain's ability to experience fictitious content that is not available in reality. The enormous worldwide success of computer games is based precisely on this ability of our brain. Phone sex, too, makes use of the ability to produce physical reactions with illusions. This does not only work for men; women can be sexually aroused with fictional content just as men are. It is a fundamental ability of our brain, which we can also use for our healing.

There is, therefore, no need for a genuine, true experience in order to have genuine, true feelings. We can examine every action and find that ultimately the imaginary part far exceeds the real part. In medicine, there are wise, free-thinking minds like MD Franz Porzsolt, director of the Institute of *Evidence Based Medicine* at the University of Ulm, who presents the opinion that ultimately any medication is a placebo and accounts for the greatest part of its efficacy from the *information* related to the use of medication.

According to our prevailing knowledge of truth and science, the high efficacy of medication must be "proven" by a study, if possible by an American one. Whereas in Africa, statements by the forefathers have the highest degree of plausibility – the credibility of the Bible is not as strong despite Christian missionary work. And in Arabic, what is written in the Koran has the highest truth. The subjectivity of truth is thus not only individually dependent, but also dependent on the superordinate *knowledge frame*, as MD Ernst Pöppel calls the plausibility frame – that is, dependent on culture.

Because of how our brains function – completely regardless of whether it is inside black, white, red, or yellow skin – every event is initially neutral. And it is the task of the respective society to figure out which fiction is the predicate *fact* and which is not. What is explained as fact becomes reality, and reality is what works. This is how simple truth is. But since your own truth is one of the most difficult things to change in life, it is not so easy with a new, positive truth.

Information has an effect on all cells.
It can make you sick or healthy.

Placebo research also shows the value of information. Information – whatever its nature – has proven to have a powerful effect on us. Everyone can confirm this from their daily life: We overhear some comment – and we are worried. The long-desired email or the call with a positive message, on the other hand, makes the soul rejoice. After an argument, the onset of anger creates a black hole for the next few hours. And because a moment spontaneously makes us laugh, the world suddenly looks friendly again, and we feel great.

Information is quick and direct: Not only does it reach our brain directly, but it also forms synapses, which in turn emit messenger substances, which regulate the entire cellular behaviour of the body. Each brain has 10 to the power of 84 synapses, that is, connectivity possibilities. In sum, there are more possibilities than there are elementary particles in the universe. It is therefore not surprising that all information, even the most casual and insignificant, and even memorised or unconsciously-acquired information, receives a specific physical reaction. As long as these reactions are within acceptable limits, we do not take notice of them. Only when we are in pain and/or given a dramatic diagnosis, do we feel the urge to consider it more closely, if we want to heal mentally with the *KUBYmethod*. It is necessary to become aware of the pathological information that has been generated and sent by the relevant synapses.

To clarify: information can heal, but it can also make you sick. Information forms synapses 400 to 4000 times faster than material intervention – i.e. injected or swallowed medication and surgery or other physiotherapeutic measures. What determines whether information – of whatever content – makes you sick or healthy? There can be no objective answer.

The same information can make one person sick and another healthy. For example, someone who has been fired has to try to find out which formulation is most effective. Which formulation is most appropriate for your own fears? If I feel so strongly affected by information such as "fired" that I become ill, then for the fastest possible recovery I have to find what anxieties are associated with it. Is there any memory of this fear of this possible downfall? It may not even be a memory, but at first only a feeling. But to fathom this is the way to healing.

This path can also be shortened by saying, for example, in a shocking situation: "I forgive the company for firing me. I give the company my love and thank it for everything it has done for me." If you can manage to not only thank it, but also express and write down this thanks, it is certainly easier for you afterwards, and perhaps will also help you get back on your feet. If the energy of life still remains clouded, and a new fulfilling job or activity is not in sight, then this course of action is not enough. Then you simply can't get around discovering the causative history (information) that nourishes your current fears.

No doubt: **information has an impact**. Since human beings are an information system – what, as we have seen, concerns their physical response to negative information – it is worth a try to reverse and generate positive responses with positive information. And the further good news is that, as you now know, the brain does not distinguish between fact and fiction; the fiction (the illusion) of positive information can be created.

Someone who has, for example, internalised the doctrine of faith: "You always get through it" or "somehow life goes on" will probably not be so violently shaken by being fired. For those who are unable to heal so quickly, have the task of researching so deeply in themselves until they have found the reason why the termination caused them to become so sick.

Those who create the hierarchy of being in their consciousness make their mind the guiding force of their life, and do not, therefore, attribute independent behaviour to their body, but consider it an expression, form, or manifestation of their mental state. If they have a stomach ache after being fired, they would recognise this as a reaction to their mental/soul illness through information and counteract it as appropriate. With positive information (such as that in the chapter "Soul Writing," chapter 3), health can sometimes be restored immediately. However, this is only possible if we have overcome our doubt about the efficacy of information and no longer give the body an independent life.

But why do most of us have such serious doubts about this kind of self-healing? Why do we not recognise our own competence? As we shall see below, this has mainly to do with how each of us sees the world.

Five human images

There are infinitely many ways to categorise the philosophies with which people experience themselves and their world. The following *five categories* allow you to determine your level of consciousness more closely. Ask yourself: What is the human image I carry in me? Without clarifying this question, further development is quite arbitrary. Let us begin with the roughest:

1. For the **material human image**, we proceed purely mechanically, for example with surgery. In 120 years, the position of a health care practitioner has risen from barber surgeons to the peak of medical interventions by means of enormously increased skills. In surgical thinking, humans resemble, as it were, a machine that can be repaired and partially replaced. Physicians speak of wearing parts, wear and tear, bad starting material, etc.

2. The more subtle consideration of humans is that of the **biochemical human image**. Through this lens, the human being resembles, in a certain way, a laboratory in which substances are formed and transformed. The input and output of cells are evaluated for this and influenced by natural and/or artificial substances. This thinking is shared by the pharmaceutical industry and most people , not only doctors.

3. On an even more subtle level, the human being is considered **an energetic being**. More than a quarter of humanity has this human image – 1.5 billion Chinese and a large number of other Asians, and now also many Westerners. According to their philosophy, humans are reduced to 4 or 5 main energies, which are in balance when the human being is healthy. Homoeopathy can also be used for this healing method, because it does not use any chemical substances, but it energetically affects humans.

4. With its higher potencies, homeopathy also goes to an even finer material level, on which the human is seen as **an information being** and nothing else is necessary for their healing than to give their body the healing information it needs. Because starting with a D 25 potency or even a D 60 potency, it can no longer be considered a substance or an energy.

   The degree of dilution of such preparations corresponds to the ratio of one drop of active substance to the water quantity of an ocean. What is effective in this case is merely the information associated with the active ingredient. This purely mental type of therapy also includes all resonance therapies, in which no substances, but only frequencies, are administered (e.g. the original Russian device *Prognos* and the devices that followed it).

   Frequencies are selected according to their information spectrum for these applications. The new homeopathy consequently works only with symbols that are painted on the patient's skin and with placebos which only transport the information content of medication. No biochemical agents are involved. Information medicine is devoid of substance and thus belongs to the category of spiritual healing.

5. The pure **spiritual-soulful (based on soul and intuition) human image**, in which no vehicle (no apparatus, no globules, nothing) is used, acts on the soul level. Here, no substances are administered – whatever potency or frequency – nor are any physical interventions or physiotherapies performed. There is no carrier for information. All necessary information is gained from the person's communication with their soul. The soul is defined as a continuum without a beginning and without an end, and the body as a temporary expression of mental condition. This human image is the basis for the *KUBYmethod.*

But what kind of human image do we commonly have? Let us look around: the abundance of available worldviews (explanatory models) is increasing at a rapid pace, as is communication. We used to wait for a letter sent by post for four weeks, and then write back at our convenience until eventually meeting to clarify the matter. Today we become anxious if a message sent via the Internet and satellite does not arrive in minutes and cannot be immediately spread across the world. The requirement to see images of events on the other side of the globe in the shortest possible time is normal nowadays. Software updates and the development of communication tools have reached a speed that leaves us breathless and makes us feel like we are constantly chasing after the latest development – this is a race we can´t win.

Despite this high density of events, the materialist image of humankind persists in our minds permanently. This view of the world always assumes an objective reality. The idea that this reality arises only from your own interpretation and your own beliefs is difficult to accept today. In the materialistic view scales can be used which precisely describe a state: weight dimensions, length measurements, colour scales, material knowledge, time measurement, etc. On the inside, however, precision is directed towards authenticity and the purely subjective perception of experiences, pain, pleasure, suffering, love, and so on.

Still criteria are much too fuzzy and imprecise. Of course materialists (at times) see the emotional side of the picture, but it makes them feel insecure. Women generally have fewer problems than men in this regard. Men are brought up to be even more focused on the materialist human image than women are. It is therefore more difficult for men than for women to embrace feelings and to make an evaluation (see the following example). The fear is too great that suddenly their tough masculine image, which has been cultivated for millennia, will suddenly collapse.

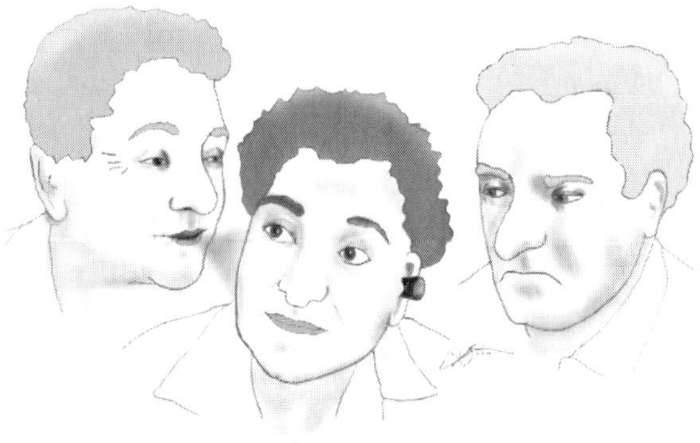

---

*"Who do I listen to?
This is my own responsibility."*

MEN ONLY

"Better not talk about it ..."

Shutting down, protecting yourself against being hurt

Both professionally or in private, most men find it very unpleasant, sometimes even horrible, to talk about personal things. Is it dangerous? If so, why? As soon as you share things, emotions come into play. And men are afraid that they cannot withstand them. What they allow themselves to do while watching football in the stands is primal behaviour and simply not practical for everyday life. Finely formulated emotionality is not in their nature.

I realise that every man is different, but in general typical behaviour patterns can always be observed. A man, for example, thinks that he is not allowed to give in to his "emotions," but must be as rational, strong, hard, and cool as possible – a deeply anchored conviction handed down over many generations.

This role is certainly changing from what it once was, but my seminars show very clearly how difficult men still suffer from this oldfashioned understanding of roles. Many of them still grew up hearing things like "Boys don't cry." "Well, you're not a girl." "Hey, you wimp, you sissy." "Tough guys know no pain." You want to be a big, strong boy." and so on. All of this, of course, has an effect on adult men.

And so we end up as a partner and a family guy and don't know how to deal with our feelings. At the most, they can be released in the stadium, but to bring them into communication, deal with them, and maybe even approve of them is a different story. Men prefer to deal with their emotions privately. Emotions can be dodged and diverted by talking about sports, alcohol, small talk, food etc. while outwardly only a pretence of confidence is shown. Many are much better at acting this way than being "effeminate". Who wants to be seen as a weakling? Feelings are fundamentally dangerous, they can make the usual order of things quite messy, and this alone makes men feel stressed. Understandably, then, men are afraid of women when they say "honey, we need to talk ..." and respond by running away.

Can this dilemma somehow be resolved? Experience shows that insight into existing behaviour hardly changes anything. No, the male gender role must be grabbed by the root – by exercising emotions! A good start for this is getting out their old childhood photos. Some men find even this too overwhelming. Women have far fewer problems confronting their baby and toddler existence, and even enjoy it. Men, on the other hand, as soon as they hear a disparaging word about themselves like "the little chicken," create an inner distance for themselves.

But it's still worthwhile to try! When you look at your early photos, you'll probably see some of the events that make you aware of how the prevailing lack of emotions developed. Suddenly you discover that you used to be a very tender, loving soul who needed to be cuddled, but you were weaned off this. This can cause tears, which you shouldn't be ashamed of. On the contrary, you now have the chance to correct this. When you see yourself as a child and remember how painful and heartless your upbringing might have been, there is the possibility of correcting this upbringing NOW. How this works and what exactly happens will be described in chapter 3.

There are various explainable models, including scientific ones, for this process to retroactively change your upbringing following the motto "it's never too late to have a happy childhood". But perhaps this is only of secondary importance for you at the moment, because you are suddenly in contact with your intuition through memories and can let it in. In doing so, you will have the experience that that what was is alive on the emotional level in the now and has an impact there. And what is in the now can also be changed *now*.

Such processes may at first be unfamiliar, but can be practised with the *KUBYmethod*. And so, step by step, it becomes possible to enter a healthy and happy reality, in which feelings also have their place. And that does not only affect emotions such as anger, rage, and pain, but also tender feelings, including those that lead to joyful tears.

Women drink medicinal teas,
men prefer antibiotics.

People who are still heavily arrested in a materialistic consciousness desperately want material intervention as pain killers. They do not consider self-healing, but ask for external help. Yet this help should not include any cause research, rather they want love, attention, anaesthesia, rest, consolation – preferably a miracle. It would be particularly great to be able to say shortly afterwards: "It was nothing." "A weak spell?" "No, only …" And then you quickly find fault with something external like the weather, air conditioning, the position of the moon, the aftermath of travelling, the food, the drink, etc.; and if there is nothing acute to be found, then it is an old story that still comes from an accident or an earlier illness, or perhaps inherited, and so on and so on … all sorts of things are considered except for self-consideration.

The change in the human image from one level of consciousness to the next represents in the individual the great, evolutionary development process of mankind. In this way, spirituality is also found in matter and is reconciled with it. This means that matter is combated, destroyed, manipulated, removed, or artificially replaced at the material, conventional medicine level of consciousness. It is only when you are "forced" to heal yourself, because all other methods have not helped, that you gain matter (the body) as a friend since you experience it as an expression of your own thinking.

If we have freed matter (the body) of pain and suffering through other thinking, **reconciliation** is accomplished. But of course not for all time, because we are constantly evolving and thus at a further stage of consciousness we are once again challenged to recognise the spiritual cause of a material symptom and to solve it spiritually. In death, we cannot escape this challenge. Previously compromises were possible, even if they were by no means purposeful. A compromise arises when resistance to knowledge of the spiritual cause cannot be overcome. Such resistances have very different reasons.

Nevertheless no resistance is pointless or blocks progressing with the *KUBYmethod*, rather it is in itself an additional task for the consciousness. **If you feel like you are standing in front of a wall** and can't go further, the wall itself is already the subject: How long and how high is the wall? How does it feel? What possibilities do you have to think about in order to overcome it? **Men usually pick up a jack-hammer, women get a rope ladder** … Play around with your resistance (no matter how it is presented) until it is overcome. Then suddenly you can see what it looks like on the other side of the wall. (Tip: Make sure you know each of these steps in writing – see the instructions in chapter 3.)

Important: do not wait until someone shows you how to overcome your resistance in your process within the framework of the *KUBYmethod*, instead take it as a challenge.

When it comes to dying, we cannot keep up our resistance of leaving the body. At exactly that point, we need an idea to keep going. In doing so, it very much helps you to see yourself (as a matter of fact, immediately) as a spiritual being, because then we don't die. If you identify with your soul, you are immortal.

The mind and soul are much more than a body. No matter how closely we examine the body: we will find neither spirit nor soul in it. But we experience the soul in intuitive states, with senses, premonitions, and feeling. Every human being therefore knows that they possess spirit and soul. These terms are not universally defined for our society today, which is why everyone defines it differently. What is important, however, is that we do not give the body a life of its own. For the body is nothing more than a tool to gain experience with which you can develop your consciousness.

Why do we find this spiritual-soulful perspective so difficult? The difficulty with the spiritual human image is due to the fact that the life of the soul does not begin with conception or birth. Usually as adults we no longer remember what we experienced before we were conceived. Yet children do so without problems. But the parents and other caregivers who have not internalised their own consciousness as a continuum do not notice it or interpret it as childish thing.

Evolution of consciousness is very slow given the forms (bodies) that express consciousness. It takes place only in relatively small leaps, even if they are subjectively experienced as revolutionary. This experience exists on every level of consciousness. For everyone their next step of consciousness is equally difficult and there is always a subsequent step for everyone. It is not a question of consciousness as a whole, but in certain areas of life. I have not yet met an enlightened person who could not develop as intensely as any other being.

Enlightened or not (yet) enlightened, ask yourself again and again: Which of the aforementioned human images makes an impact on me? It is worth taking a crystal clear position here in order not to be deceived by yourself and then perhaps to complain about the fact that self-healing doesn't work? Simply try it out, for example with the well-known subject of annoyance. If you encounter it with the spiritual-soulful human image, you will find that it is above all a question of interpretation.

Each of us is confronted with minor or major annoyances in everyday life. Here, too, you can relax a lot more when you realise: I am never annoyed by the reason I think, because all annoyance is (simply) an attempt to justify my own interpretation. If I change the interpretation, the annoyance does not apply, because now there is no reason for it – even if the event remains the same. The reason for the annoyance cannot have been in the event itself, but only in the interpretation (in the evaluation, the judgement), in how I thought about the event.

If I want to justify my interpretation, I want to make it come true and thus create a seemingly real reason for my annoyance, especially for events that I interpret as hostile. With my interpretation of the event, I can give my own annoyance so much justification (so much legitimisation) that I can even attack the supposed enemy.

In this way I abuse an event to justify my interpretation (my annoyance about the supposed attack on me). This thought system can only recognise (or interpret) an attack because it is thinking about attacking itself. A thought system that includes the idea of an "attack" with which I interpret the event seems more important to me than thoughts such as peace, health, happiness, and harmony, with which I could also interpret the event. I do not need to create a new event for this interpretation. There do not have to be any new events that I have no influence on. All I need is my thought system to be ready to let go of what I justify as hostile interpretations of events. All it takes is to think differently – so that the spiritual possibilities can be expanded.

Why this point is so important will become clear in the next chapter. Because it is not enough to just want to be healthy – we have to *choose health too!*

2

Choosing to be healthy

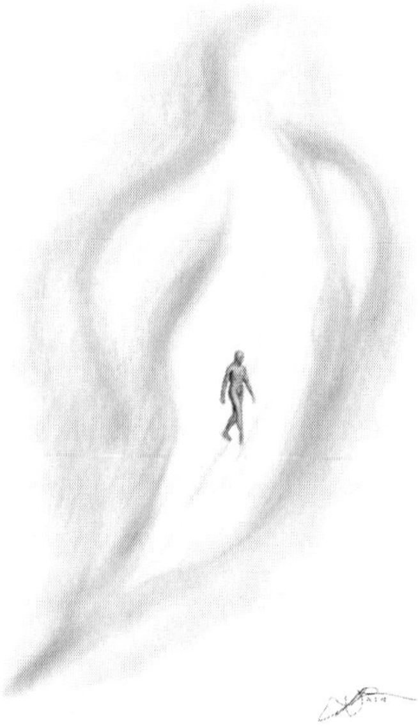

"We are a soul with a body, not a body with a soul."

The soul wants truthfulness and not profiteering

Humans are self-healing beings. If this were not so, the many people I personally met when they were considered incurable and who are now healthy – as I am – would not exist. Every person is equipped in such a way that they have their own direct connection with the universe. Even though this connection is not activated for most people, the base is nevertheless available to everyone and can be used at any time. No external conditions have to be fulfilled; you will become aware of this at the latest after reading this book. But that needs a decision – to be made by you, and right now!

In a similar way, even the current health system requires this of us: the enlightened patient is supposed to not only heal himself, but also the health system. If you want to remain fit as you get older, as health insurance companies and politics want you to, you need to take responsibility for your own health. Patients' rights need to be strengthened for this, and "the old authoritarian relationship between doctors and patients should be transformed into a partnership." Whether it is the government, medical organisations, or health insurance companies, all of them are talking about the self-determination right of the patients. Has something actually changed in the public consciousness? Patients no longer want to feel like they are being treated by those above them. Instead they want to be enlightened and asked what treatment the doctor wants to use for them. Most doctors need to get used to this.

But in what matters should the patients actually have a say? They do not know anything about medicine. There are now self-help groups and the Internet, but what they find there are only medical considerations that do not promote their self-healing skills, but often only frighten them more. As a result, as long as the prognoses cannot be expected to be hazardous to life, most of them remain passive and swallow what they are prescribed.

Why is this the case? The conception of ourselves does not allow for any other alternative. We live in a materialistic age after all. We do not learn to communicate with our souls. Thus, we can no longer approach the causative mental impulse and operate exclusively on symptom control. This is where our current medicine is specialised. This health care system, however, now costs a lot of money, which people can barely afford. The non-wage labour costs even consume the companies' profits and the capital migrates to low-wage countries where there are no such high health insurance contributions. If we calculate the reason why Germany as a place of business is at risk, then it is the medications included in the non-wage labour costs. Our health concept, therefore, has an impact on the entire economy and on all employment.

A health concept that consciously works with self-healing would be a benefit for everyone. Still, as we have already seen in chapter 1, the whole agenda is primarily a question of philosophy. For this reason, medical practitioners who want to be part of the solution must also be prepared to change the way they look at themselves. It is certainly not easy for someone who has studied medicine to see humans as a spiritual being, and physicality merely as an expression or reflection of mental consciousness processes. However, more and more thoughtful doctors have now succeeded in doing this.

Progress means better differentiating of what exists. Therefore what exists does not disappear, on the contrary – the new emerges from it and therefore does not have to be attacked as something menacing, strange. Yet progress often appears to many as bad, because it puts what already exists off balance. However, if you look at this more closely, then what exists is also not in balance, as the doctors themselves admit, it is only what is familiar. For example, if every year thousands die from the unwanted side effects of pills, it cannot be described as an equilibrium, but at most as something to which we have become accustomed, which we have, so to speak, accepted out of incapacity. But the fate of all those who die from this backwardness should be an invitation to us to want to learn something that extends our possibilities of healing.

The need for substantial progress is evident in view of the problems that our health care system faces. In addition, as already mentioned, this system is increasingly difficult to finance and impoverishes millions of people. Given this urgency, medicine and science should no longer be able to afford to earn money and recognition by taking on tasks (research projects) that others have long ago solved.

However, since we are not interested in solutions that question one's business and high privileges, such solutions are considered unscientific. The dogma of "scientific" establishes an ideological wall against philosophies which are far closer to life than what is called scientific materialism.

What does the patient do if the doctor cannot help them with their seeming scientific view of humans? Most of them then go to a healing practitioner or homeopath, and then – if they do not find a cure there either – many people dare to visit a healer. But even a healer often cannot provide a cure.

Those who still do not give up and do not want their lives to end in illness, then perhaps discover the concept of self-healing, true to the motto: "help yourself, otherwise nobody will help you". This development from conventional medicine to self-healing represents the gradual change of the human image in the consciousness of the patient. As already mentioned, this development often springs from need and without consciousness of the philosophy on which the different methods are based. As a patient, you only realise that the "vehicles" of the individual methods become more subtle from stage to stage, up to pure thinking without any auxiliary means.

Once you reach the point where you understand that you are a spiritual being, you can do so with the same comfortable attitude you had at the conventional medicine level, without self-responsibility. Just as pills were somehow used to eliminate the disease, a divine energy is now being absorbed which will also eliminate the disease. The mental cause of the illness remains hidden in the subconscious, at least if you do not have the self-competence to become conscious of it. Prayers remain just as mystical as pills. The side effects of prayers and pills mean dependency in both cases.

Healthy without Medicine, on the other hand, means freedom through causative self-healing. That is, we recognise not only the spiritual cause of the problem or illness, but also the message that we gain from the disease or problem for our development (see chapter 3). In this way, we recognise the high value of any challenge that is a disease or a major life problem. Ultimately we are grateful to the suffering that forced us to evolve.

Each one of us is born with a whole spectrum of feelings. Even if we feel predominantly selfish, we know other sides of ourselves. The question of which side or which aspects of our emotional spectrum we are encouraging is a question of consciousness.

However, as long as self-healing is not an option for our own well-being, no need for self-initiative, we are dependent on people who we believe know better than ourselves, which can be good or bad. This vision of always relying on a professional to stay healthy and happy has become the biggest business of all time. Accordingly this awareness is anchored deeply in everyone, which is why we accept working for it daily without protest. This fact is only known by a few. This business is based on the automatic and compulsory procurement of funds in the form of health insurance contributions, which are deducted from most people's wages without them being able to do anything about it. Self-employed people are also now compulsorily insured. Both groups together constitute 97% of the working population.

It is also done for people who are not sick, supposedly with solidarity for the others who are sicker than they can afford to be. In reality this compulsory system only serves the industry and its representatives (i.e. doctors) to be able to collect money at all times, even from those who are healthy. This alleged solidarity can therefore only be claimed within the framework of the prevailing ideology (the bio-chemical, mechanical human image). Otherwise the pharmaceutical industry could not stay in business. Thus there is no question of freedom of choice.

Of course this is at the expense of the patients. They are often so weakened and intimidated that they can no longer stand up for their right and look for alternatives. They simply let themselves be overruled – regardless of the costs, even if they do not get necessarily healthier, but perhaps even worse, through many treatments.

Why are people willing to accept such a burden? It is **business based on fear**. This business works because anxiety is based on a philosophy that – to reemphasize – defines humans as material beings. The gigantic health sector is therefore only a by-product of the ruling materialism. But it contributes very strongly in keeping people trapped in this fear. The fear that underlies this materialistic image of mankind captures everyone sooner or later automatically, even those who earn their money with this human image.

Feel the fear inside that overcomes you if you are not insured. To feel this fear, you do not have to be sick, but only have to have internalised the mechanical or biochemical view of life. Your entire identity depends on such a materialistic human image in which the soul has no place. In contrast, if you identify with your soul (the individualised Great Spirit) and you get your health and happiness from this, then you cannot be afraid. Without fear in the materialistic human image, the whole business of managing disease would not emerge, and things would be much better for everyone.

A health system that defies the freedom and dignity of man cannot continue to exist. The expense and the number of victims are too great, and in the long run nobody can be happy and joyful with the materialistic human image. Every human being wants to be happy, which is why I am firmly convinced that the materialistic image is changing at an exponential pace.

The liberating factor in this transformation process of the human image is that we are not dependent on external conditions. Without this social change taking place, we can already free ourselves from this materialistic system because no one can forbid our self-healing. Nor can our own well-being be ultimately prohibited. The difficulty of this process consists solely in overcoming our own beliefs. It is never too early to be your own boss, and this can be put into practice immediately.

Real and fundamental **progress in our health care system** would therefore require that our society begins to train *intuition*. Our entire education system – from kindergarten to schools and professional training to university – has to date been focused on training the rational side, the left hemisphere. But with reason or what is called awakening awareness, we do not achieve our own wisdom and competence. If we want to heal ourselves and thus further develop the full expression of humanity, we need the resource of *intuition*. For this, we must also begin to train our right brain hemisphere. Please read more in the next section.

Intuition – the royal road to knowledge

Intuition is our most valuable resource. We can equate it with our soul. Every being (including humans), both men and women, have intuition. As already mentioned, women generally have a better relationship with their intuition than men, which is socially conditioned. Men are supposed to work logically and not listen to their gut. In this way, men deal more easily with constraints. But someone who listens to his soul is not so easily put under pressure. He knows that he isn't doing any favours to his health, which no one can replace.

We learn intuition most effectively by self-healing, because it does not work with our materialistic, purely rational consciousness. In self-healing processes, we sense every progress physically or experience healing through a happy reality that we create ourselves. We learn to use our intuition to solve any kind of problem – whether it be for a relationship, money, work, or a physical problem, or the ability to be in the right place at the right time, like free animals. We need a lot of flexibility and sense of urgency for this, and sooner and more often. The resource of intuition is therefore far too valuable to be allowed to perish.

MEN ONLY

"I've got it under control."

Sense of responsibility, feasibility

The main thing is being organised! This makes an impression, it gives others a good feeling, it creates trust which signals: "With me, you can be secure, you can rely on me, I have everything under control." Men are quick to accept this attitude and like to identify with such an image. No wonder, because much of this was already given to them in their education and later gives them the appropriate recognition. If an unforeseen situation arises, a bigger problem, this attitude is taken up whether it is true or not, but either way, a "real man" acts as though everything is fine. What is, on the one hand, a praiseworthy survival tactic, can, on the other hand, constitute a serious danger when it comes to health.

Why? Because men might deal with a disease as objectively as they have learnt to organise their life. This means, however, that they block access to their intuition, that is, to their soul. But only via their soul can they arrive at the cause, i.e. the *root* cause of a disease – on a factual-rational level this is more problematic.

A factual attitude towards oneself or people close to you in the case of illness often begins to stifle emerging anxieties and fears in your core with all that reason has to offer. Men are, so to speak, seeking the rational solution, that is, the solution of medicine or of the bio-chemical, materialistic, mechanical human image. Men feel responsible and want to do everything they can to get the job done. They firmly believe, at least, in what is possible on the path known to them, even if this often proves to be an error.

This thinking is quite obvious, because men are more familiar with the left side of their brain, the rational half. Their profession is often one on the rational side of things. They are accustomed, for example, to dealing with machines, figures, and facts. They are convinced that most things, maybe even *everything*, is feasible when it has to be.

What initially sounds like pronounced self-confidence, however, can easily tilt into self-assessment if the feasibility is attributed solely to materially shaped factors. This means, of course, that all investigations that can be conceived of are agreed on. Any treatment, however exhausting it may be, is tried out ("My doctor said ..."). Numbers and statistics are sought which give the disease X and the symptom Y this or that chance. And, of course, during all this, they keep working so they can prove everything is working out as planned. Many men need this feeling – or rather, this illusion – because they simply cannot cope with an open-ended future.

If you are familiar with this, and perhaps because of a current situation you are subliminally having more and more doubts and concerns that you can ignore less and less, this is the opportunity to take countermeasures in other ways. No, you do not have to give up reason, but use it to enter into another process of consciousness. And this begins with telling others about your needs and worries! No matter how soberly and factually you do it, talk to someone you trust. If the other person listens well, you will probably find the right words for your feelings as well.

Once you talk with others about your mental state and your worries, you are given the opportunity to reflect. And this creates a new awareness of pain, disease, the deepest human fear of what will be.

If the step towards a more intensive exchange with others is still too risky, the conversation can first start with yourself: In *soulwriting* you will get the ideal "sparring partner" for this … Give it a try: if you not only give your mind the privilege, but also allow your soul and thus your intuition to speak up, an increase in consciousness will occur. In this way, you may not feel the pressure to have everything under control so strongly. You will learn to feel and to be able to trust your feelings more and more. This also promotes trust in your subjective truth. Humans, and thus you yourself, are not just a meat sack with a few bones, hair and teeth, rather there is a spirit standing over us – with no beginning and no end.

So give control back to your spirit, because the body is 100% subordinate to the mind! Mental health is also physical health. At this level, you decide how you and the people close to you are doing – because it is about peace, love, security, and recognition. And these values are not under control, they are not "feasible", but they want to be lived. Your intuition will be and remain a valuable compass and reliable companion.

But how do we succeed in creating a new reality through our free spirit? A good example is the actor. Actors are always in the same body, but they consistently play other beings. Their bodies, their matter, in the case of a good actor always seems to represent precisely what they mentally imagine. You can also use this technique for any kind of problem-solving, including on the path to becoming healthy.

It is always about the hurdle to change from material identity to spiritual identity. If the spiritual identity of your being is self-evident, then you can choose the role you want to play. Including such roles that appear to be foolhardy or ridiculous at first. The more you accept your role, the more obvious you will fill it in your mind – whether beggars or kings, whether murderers or saints, whether politicians or family fathers, esteemed employees or well paid workers: everyone is everyone. With the "as-if" attitude, you can slip into any role and thereby gain feelings that you did not even know of in the entity you are "playing" or believe yourself to be. It is, for example, astonishing to slip into the skin of a blind person as someone who can see, even if it is only for a few hours. After doing so, you will gain an experience and reverence for blindness that no word, text, or film could ever convey.

The fact that we are spiritual beings does not mean, however, that we are good beings. It merely means that everything that is conceivable in the mind can be materialised with enough energy, and thus turned into reality. In the desolate state of humankind, we can see that what is conceived of with energy is also realised.

People have not yet realised that we can change our role at any moment. The material conditions serve only as props for the selected role. And the props do not determine the role, rather the role determines the props. Example: If someone is leading a terrible marriage in poverty, then that is also a role that they have accepted and fulfilled. If they were aware of the fact that they are a spiritual being, they could sit down and write down a different role for themselves, which they would rather play and, in doing so, determine how their fellow players behave. It does, of course, take work to conceive of such a role, and consider each player's role and which props go with it. But it is the best way to get rid of their misery.

Let us learn to think holistically and put our intuition above reason, so that we reach our own wisdom.

Consider: What props do you need to fully take on the role of a happy, healthy person? And: You need a precise script for the creation of your role so you actually "learn to walk". I will describe how to proceed with this in the next chapter.

Always remember: **The body (matter) is subordinate to the mind.** This means you are able to realise your new reality. If the mind was not the boss, the new reality would not be created, and the law of action (karma) would not be carried out. The spiritual freedom to think about what you want is the basis for the freedom of life with the possibility to determine your destiny. This also applies to life in the future. The idea becomes quite self-evident if you acknowledge the continuum of the spirit I talked about in chapter 1.

All spiritual healing depends on the credibility of a new reality. How can it be achieved? Since on the soul or intuitive level everything happens now, there are no space and time barriers on the mental level. That is why you always formulate the transcription or imagination of a new reality in the present form and in literal speech – just as we do when reconstructing the pain image.

To emphasise it again: **Reality is what has an effect**! At the level of intuition, we experience enough situations in which reality is a complete illusion, but one that still works.

The *KUBYmethod* presents us with a task that is gigantic. You can start with it immediately without needing prerequisites, but you are never done with it either. If we understood how much energy was needed to develop the resource of ratio, we would realise what new dimensions are opening up through the resource of intuition. We must discover these dimensions again.

Ratio was not always the focus of our discussion. A long time ago, the Arabs, for example, had developed the structuring thought system of mathematics. In Europe, we were still quite intuitive – today it is the other way round. In the development of human consciousness, there is, therefore, a constant, large-scale pendulum movement between reason and intuition – that is, between training the right and left hemispheres. If we have had enough experience with one-sided extremes, there is hope that one day we will become holistic people who are both rational and intuitive.

That is why I am committed to promoting the training of intuition (ideally from a young age!) with the clear position that this should not be at the expense of reason. Both optimally complement each other. The *KUBYmethod* will be of interest to all those who are struggling on the path of pure reason, or those who already live with this limit, such as "incurable", "forever chronically ill," "permanently genetically handicapped," or "victimised" people etc. Everyone has the urge for freedom and dignity. Even these two motives are sufficient to extend our scope for action. With the *KUBYmethod*, you receive a health philosophy that broadens the boundaries of the rational, materialistic approach and finds areas where freedom and dignity are fully utilised.

Our soul is patient, so incredibly patient – until it becomes unbearable by making the previous unhealthy life concept massively physically noticeable. But we should not let it come to that. Let us learn to understand our **soul interest** early and realise that the soul does not have to be heard through painful experiences. We want to leave our bodies one day healthy and happy. If we do not accept the contact with our soul in this life, it will make itself known in the next life. At some point, we will learn to listen to it. Now would be the best time.

Recognising and using your own competence

When people are asked what is most important to them in life, about 80% of the population say "health". At the same time, however, they have the lowest competence on this issue. This means that despite all appeals from health politicians, people are not able to take on their own responsibility – they simply do not know how to. This is also not possible with the universally propagated, dominant human image. Our biggest project, therefore, should be to change our human image that we carry within ourselves. As already mentioned, it is materialistic in our era. But we notice more and more that with this image many goals cannot be achieved, such as the goal of being healthy and happy and also die as such.

Self-responsibility needs competence to let deeds follow. With the consciousness of being a mechanical and biochemical being, you would have to be a doctor yourself to exercise self-responsibility. But surgeons do not operate on themselves, and doctors are just as sick as their patients. Truly lived self-responsibility needs a human image with which you can be your own boss and not be plagued by transient anxieties.

If you consider your materialistic, biochemical being only one step more finely, that is, less coarsely, then we have already gotten to emotions – and they lead us immediately away from medicine. For example, something like the fear of dying, with which medicine is constantly driving its business, is not a medical matter, but a purely philosophical one. This is precisely why it is necessary to change their human image. If you have a human image in which there is no reason to be afraid of dying, you can no longer be blackmailed by medicine.

Philosophy chooses the human image with which we move through life. **We need a philosophy according to which we not only live well, but also die well.** But this should not happen only when death is imminent, rather right now when there is still time to actively work on our own transformation. You do not need to wait until you are in pain. The advantages of a more subtle to spiritual human image can also be reaped without illness. You do not have to be incurable to be forced by fear of death to expand your consciousness because all material possibilities for intervention have been exhausted.

By changing your human image, you can begin immediately. If you want to change, you must first know where it is. Otherwise, it does not feel the change and does not know where to start. Perhaps it is not even clear to you through which glasses you should look at the world, that is, what consciousness you currently possess. This can usually only be seen in retrospect. It is only when you practice a new behaviour that you become aware of what consciousness you had before. If, however, we want to consciously develop further, it is worthwhile to first assess our actual state.

Simply take a look in your medicine cabinet. Everything that is in it represents the materialistic biochemical human image – no matter how spiritual you are otherwise oriented. All these medicines have meaning only in that at least a part of your own thinking believes in them, if you see yourself or your cells as a kind of chemical laboratory in which substances are mixed and combined to regulate your condition. This human image serves the belief that thought processes (mental activities) and chemical processes could be separated from each other.

In addition to this idea, it usually also includes the assumption that chemical processes are superior to mental processes (thinking), that is, that the chemistry in the body is independent of thinking. This gives the materialistic and the corresponding chemical human image an enormous position in the hierarchy of your own being. But if the thinking of chemistry is to be subordinated, who would be the boss of chemistry?

Every expansion of consciousness requires courage, and this is again a question of **character**. Our character is shaped by the world and human image that represents our education, which we enjoyed at home, at school, and afterwards. However, with the dominant human image which our education teaches, we fail evolution. This leads to many victims. But you do not have to be a part of this when developing your consciousness.

And there are infinitely many ways. The most commonly chosen way is the one via your own pain. Theoretically, it is difficult to achieve another concept of belief. Everyone has a vehement interest in being freed from their pain. If they also want to preserve their dignity and freedom, this means freeing *yourself* from your pain yourself. But some people get to this point only when others can no longer help them with their approach (philosophy), and the pain can no longer be accepted. At that moment, perhaps the realisation dawns that it could be or even must be about philosophy if all the paths that have been taken so far do not lead to fortune.

Some believe yes, if they have a disease like many others, then the treatment should be the same. The fact that every human being is a unique being and therefore needs a different treatment, which must take place according to their development, is usually neglected. If in the mental image of the human being you consider illness not as a misfortune, chance, or an error in the system but as a "development aid", it is only a question of hearing the message which would give the illness, the problem for your own development.

A very important aspect of this message, however, is to be sure to correct your way of life because your current approach hurts and causes problems. The philosophy of the spiritual human image is that simple. Pain or pressing problems show you that you are not on the right track to the summit of happiness (or rather to the summit of *your* happiness), because there is not only one for all people. A summit platform cannot be that big. It is always about your personal summit of happiness, and it is as unique as you are.

To emphasise again, there are no general diseases. Everyone has their own individual, personal development. Since this never stops, we cannot stop, or we will get sick. If we continue our development, we will get well again (until we lose our way again the next time). The more attentively we encourage our own development to our summit of happiness, the more harmless the disease (course corrections) that we suffer.

WOMEN ONLY

"But somebody has to do it!"

The caring tic, dominance in the mantle

It begins at an early age with dolls: they are cuddled and cared for, proudly presented, and kept a careful eye on – "mummy" has to do everything. The years of practised child care, this "learning for life", of course, continues into adulthood. "Taking care of it yourself" is transferred to different everyday areas, it becomes your self-purpose, a life-spirit. Women like to – both privately and professionally – make sure that everything is running properly. Of course, exceptions always prove the rule, but most women unerringly follow this caring instinct and their ability to act empathically and forward-looking. This may be wise for evolutionary reasons and still makes sense. So far, so good.

But it becomes problematic if this feminine ability goes beyond the goal, and if the altruistic motifs carry other, disguised aspects with them. Those who think they have to take care of everything can take a closer look at their motives and find out what is possibly behind them. You do not have to wait until you are dissatisfied, frustrated, and exhausted.

If you are in a similar situation, simply ask yourself the following questions: How do I feel when I have to take more breaks? – Do I get uneasy at the idea that someone else is concerned about the house and the garden, the professional project, the organisation of the planned party, the children, relatives who are perhaps in need of care? – Is someone really expecting me to be there for them around the clock, or do I just assume it? – or the like.

Others, on the other hand, thrive on being fully useful to others, they are energised by it, and it never occurs to them that they might be overdoing it; at least as long as tensions arise in their environment until their own soul thwarts an unpleasant symptom, or until open conflicts arise which make their own commitment very hard to keep to.

Ask yourself: Is my level of commitment the right degree for myself and others? – Do I overtax my fellow people and myself with my power? – Do I perhaps cut one piece of freedom for another because I think I know best about what is good for them? – or the like.

Compassion and selflessness are certainly indispensable qualities for harmonious cohabitation. They can, however, become a trap if they conceal claims to power, which are so to say enforced via the back door: "Give it to me, I'll do it." What sounds so helpful can also reveal dominance to make others dependent. It is the thought: "Without me, it will go wrong and end in chaos." Another popular saying is "Is that how you thank me for everything I've done for you?" Those who wield the moral club must ask the question of whether they are really acting selflessly, or, if their desire for dominance is concealed by a mantle …

This described behaviour is of course also to be found in many men. But women are generally more caring, and so they pack their egoistical interests into such an early-established virtue. Too much care can constrict others and trap them. And those who make "sacrifices" too often run the risk of forgetting themselves – their own needs, goals, and dreams. Presumably the soul has already sent a few signals by this time, but they have been deliberately ignored. After all, a "good person" has things to do ... Some people do not wake up properly until they get sick. This is the last alarm signal, however, that "Mother Theresas" should hear before prioritising their own needs instead.

With *soulwriting*, you can certainly learn more about your motivations and about what shortcomings your selflessness in life may lead to. But this first requires a decision: one for yourself! If you consider yourself indispensable, primarily for others, and yourself at most in second or third place, this is the most important prerequisite for change and self-healing. It begins with the courage to think differently. With this, and with your intuition, you will find out a lot about your life. Be open to giving yourself more affection. Let care be taken – not only for others, but also for yourself. Take care of yourself!

If we pay particular attention, we will die healthy and happy because we are looking forward to our next tool (the body), with which we can once again have very different experiences than with our current tool. We love new experiences and know that with a male body we can only have male experiences. If a man wants a woman's experience, he has to leave his body. And the more precisely he wants his next experience, the easier he will die.

I myself, for example, quite consciously **refused paying a pension scheme, because I am not financing an ailing time**. As soon as the current tool that is my body has worn out, I will give it up and create a new one according to my wishes. Last time this change worked out very well. I have only experienced beautiful things, even falling off the roof was ultimately WONDER-ful. Because I was neither without consciousness nor depressed for a second. I did not react to the diagnosis of being in a "wheelchair for life". A few people did not like that, but I did not react to it. Although I never knew how it would go for me, I consciously left it open. And, lo and behold – after a year I was able to leave the paraplegic clinic on two legs and only filmed spiritual films through which I myself could gain many spiritual insights. To this day, I live from raising awareness through films, seminars, and lectures. This was already my intention at my last death. And in the next life? We will see …

What about you? What development does your illness, your problem (let us say "project" instead) ask of you? Write down the last time you made a decision using your soul. Your soul knows your whole way to the summit of your happiness. However, if you do not follow your soul, it will send you messages – and then it is only a question of how well you listen. As loud as the soul must call to you, as strong is the suffering you are experiencing. So listen to your soul again to get healthy. What you will find is always only yours, your very own. No matter how many other people (beings) were in the same situation, this is all about your subjective truth, and it needs to be cured. Do not waste time with general interpretations and explanations. Once you have healed what has personally hurt you, you are embedded in love, that is, in the **harmonic vibration of the universe.**

Albert Einstein said, "God does not throw dice." He said that there is no coincidence in this universe. The law of cause and effect applies universally and invariably. No one is "accidentally" ill or gets into an accident accidentally. The cause of your illness always lies in a conflict which has not yet been resolved, which, incidentally, often does not even have to take place in this life, but occurred in a former one. But do not worry: if you trust your soul, this conflict regains consciousness through corresponding inner images.

We must not allow reason to be wiped away or prohibit it for ideological reasons. Of course, it can happen – and unfortunately very often – that we do not recognise the cause of an effect (immediately). To assert there was no cause for the phenomenon (effect) is therefore nonsense. It must then be researched until we arrive at a decisive conclusion.

Materialists also know and accept the law of cause and effect, but they do not accept any spiritual causes. Their thinking begins only when something has already materialised. Spiritual causes are negated or relegated to the field of speculation. The materialist argument says that some people have a better immune system than others. In the scientific sense, however, the "immune system" is just as unprovable a category as the "soul." Both terms are merely hypotheses. To prove them, a causality is presented that confirms itself, because it is based on nothing that could be perceived with our five senses. So it does not matter whether something exists objectively (there is no such thing anyway), but only whether the concept offers structure, and thus a scope for action with which certain development is possible.

As I have already made clear in this book, in the development of healing the term “soul” offers much more possibilities than the term “immune system”. Because the soul possesses many more faculties; it is also easier to communicate with the soul than with the immune system because the soul can be personalised.

As a spiritual being you are part of the Great Spirit, that is, part of the universe or God, thus, you are a divine being. All of us are, and therefore we are not separated from the all embracing spirit, even when we feel alone. Alone means that we are with the *universe*, thus alone.

Even if we agree with what has been said so far: under pressure (illness can exert great pressure), we mostly fall back into our habitual, materialistic human image. We hope for mechanical, biochemical measures, and finally, we ask (again) for them, hoping to alleviate our suffering.

In order to deal with pain and the suffering in self-responsibility, it would be important to first completely clarify that everything that materialises has a spiritual origin in such a state. In order to deal with pain and anomalies independently and competently, we need a credible, convincing philosophical basis, with which we can again remove ourselves from our suffering by spiritual means. The synapses in the brain are formed by the personal belief system. As long as this is not strong enough, the formation of synapses remains hesitant, and you wait for the physical effect of mental work in vain.

You should, therefore, look at the core of your conviction. With the *KUBYmethod*, it is about making yourself your first consultant. Because no one knows you better than yourself you develop a systematic approach that will take you to your deepest knowledge of yourself. For this system, among other things, the structuring concept of the "soul" is used, as you have already come to know in this book.

A man who is moving his pelvis to the music and a woman who is speaking her mind in front of many people are steps of evolution which let the soul rejoice.

As soon as you acknowledge and use this model, you will notice that there is something else that is part of the process of self-healing: the desire to be happier now and immediately, and to take responsibility for it. At the same time, you recognise your own competence in an outstanding way. Such decisions can be made in any position. They do not need any special circumstances, even if you have already completely given yourself into the hands of the materialists.

How can such a decision be expressed? Some examples: Formulate what you want to be: say it out loud and write it down. You can also sing the decision instead of just speaking it; you can paint it instead of writing it, and you can dance it instead of just singing: "I am a spiritual, self-loving, and self-healing being." With such an affirmation, you give your change of consciousness a push that will inspire more ideas.

You can find out more about the manifold possibilities of communicating with your soul in the next chapter.

3

The KUBYmethod

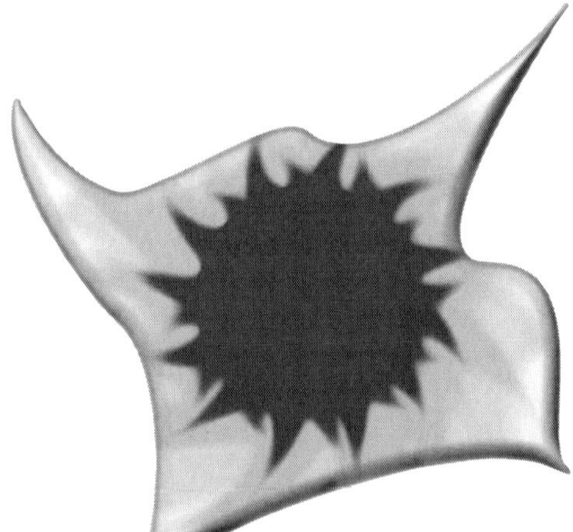

"Every cell radiates and is intelligent."

Soul writing

In this chapter, you will now learn more about the practice of self-healing and will also be able to gain practical experience. A central element of *the KUBYmethod* is *soulwriting*®, the application of which is presented in detail from page 91 onwards.

In addition, other elements are also important so that the process can be divided into three stages:

- Deep breathing (preparing the alpha state)
- Root cause research (intuitive, written)
- Soulwriting (chronological, including resolution of the pain image and its rewriting)

Deep breathing

The deep breathing exercise is the ideal preparation for soulwriting. This allows you to create what is called *the alpha state*: This is the state between awakened consciousness and sleeping consciousness, a kind of twilight state in which the activity of the brain has a frequency range between 7 and 14 Hz. If the process is getting too much for you, you can also use the following exercise on occasion to take a conscious break: before doing so, make sure you will not be interrupted for some time, have pen and paper ready (or an electronic writing instrument), and then it starts:

Place a hand relaxed and loosely on your abdomen with your thumb on your belly button. When inhaling, your hand on your lower abdomen should rise. Once the lower abdomen is filled like a balloon, but not too tight, let the air escape audibly through your slightly opened mouth. In order to feel the air column, you can "squeeze" the lower abdomen with your hand, if necessary abruptly, if this connection between the abdomen and the open valve (your mouth) is not yet working well. You recognise this by the fact that your chest and even your shoulders move as you inhale. When **breathing deeply**, this area remains completely calm and relaxed.

If necessary, loosen the clothing around your waist and hips so that your breathing can flow freely and unhindered. Do not cross your arms or legs. It is helpful if you imagine that you are sucking in air through the soles of your feet. This will make you feel more grounded and directs the air better to your lower abdomen.

Regardless of what you are dealing with at the moment, keep your mind disciplined for conscious breathing; breathe audibly to do this. Breathe calmly and slowly without straining yourself. With this relaxed breathing, exhalation often takes longer than inhalation. When your abdomen is filled well but comfortably, the air does not stop, rather, it is immediately exhaled in a relaxed way. It is best to close your eyes or unfocus your gaze and concentrate on your breathing. This is easier when you breathe out loud, because the brain identifies with the exhalation via your hearing and is not distracted by other thoughts. After three or four of these slow, deep breaths, you will notice your brain frequency slows and leaves the range of reason at over 15 hertz.

But make sure that the frequency does not fall below 7 hertz, because then you will fall asleep – and then there is no more soulwriting. When doing this exercise, it is important that the question as to the cause of the project be raised out loud (at least your lips should move) after the adjustment of deep breathing. Then write down everything that comes to mind. As soon as any phenomenon, image, concept, statement, or word is on the paper, question it. Concentrate on the feeling that emanates from your writing. That one word makes you more concerned than another. Take the concern as a guide. There is no reason not to include this deep breathing in the process several times if the process confuses you and you need rest.

Cause analysis

As already mentioned in chapter 2, intuition is the ideal way to realisation, because with it we reach areas to which we have no rational access. If we want to use our intuition not only spontaneously and unconsciously, then we need a method. Just as for rational procedures, there are also certain rules for the intuitive approach. They are part of a questioning technique that is used both *in my soul conversations®* as well as in soulwriting®. The exact instructions for this are given at the end of the book.

Defining your project: before imagining new realities with our intuition that should make us healthy and happy, we must first know what has made us sick and unhappy. In this respect, we know that there must be a precise cause for each symptom (problem/project). Rationally, it is hardly possible for us to recall the causative event, but intuitively it can be achieved – if we proceed methodologically. Ensure that you are undisturbed for a while, pick up your pen and paper (or sit at the PC) and get started:

The causative research should only be led by internal questions, i.e. those that arise from your intuition (e.g. "Why am I always so dizzy when I …? Where is it dizzy? Who makes me dizzy?" etc.). External questions are not included because they lead to abstraction and to a meta-level (e.g. "Dizziness is a widespread illness – so is it chronic if …?"). With internal questions, we allow ourselves to perceive spontaneously dormant images, sounds, and sensations and to question them in writing. Our conversation partner is our own, individualised soul. It is possible to personalise as many beings as possible (e.g. living or deceased, organs, cells, beings from inner images/dreams, spiritual beings, etc.) for soul conversations. External questions lead us away from the arising images/information instead of condensing them. Internal questions stay within the context of inner logic.

Symptom description: start your research with a description of your symptom or problem (project). For this to be successful it is crucial that this is not a medical description, but a sensed phenomenon. Often an "as if …" formulation helps here: "My … (symptom) feels as if … " Scientific descriptions (particularly Latin terms) contribute little to the healing process because they lead away from the soul.

It is certainly helpful to have an accurate diagnosis which describes what is not in order purely technically, physically, and objectively. But how the symptom feels is essential for the causative research. It is best to use adjectives that are automatically based on unconscious and repressed content. It is important to write it down immediately – even if it is not a meaningful or "only" spontaneous description, which will not be understood until later.

Tracing it back: as soon as you have these words in front of you on paper, ask yourself where you know the term or feeling from. How old is it? What experience could it be related to? When reason switches on in such moments and these thoughts are devalued as pure fantasy or even nonsense, it is ignored. Reason takes a break now. It is helpful if it simply stays *quiet* now. What is required in this process is intuition, and many things can remain very unclear at first. All "buts" are decisively cut off!

You do not listen, do not pay attention to them, but follow the pictures, words, feelings, colours, sounds, etc. that come up in response to the questions. Of course, reason will interfere again and assert: "This is all stupidity, you're imagining it," and so on and so forth. This whispering, however, does not interest us – at least not when we are about to get to know our soul. (For most people this is new territory anyway.) If in such situations you feel that nothing at all is arising, write that down. If you cannot put reason to rest, you can also write down what it has to say. After that, after a few filled lines, there is time and space for the soul to get on board. Reason always says the same thing anyway, and if you have written this down, it has done enough.

Chronological soulwriting

After you have traced the cause with the help of your intuition, the actual *soulwriting* begins. There the entire process is traversed from the cause via the impact to the solution of the problem by creating a new reality.

You can of course do this writing at any time, anywhere, but it is particularly effective in the alpha condition described above. Night hours have proved to be particularly effective. If you want to revise a topic, simply drink a lot in the evening, so you wake up during the night. But from experience, this is usually not necessary. Because your process is already beginning to work through the intent in the subconscious, you will wake up completely by yourself.

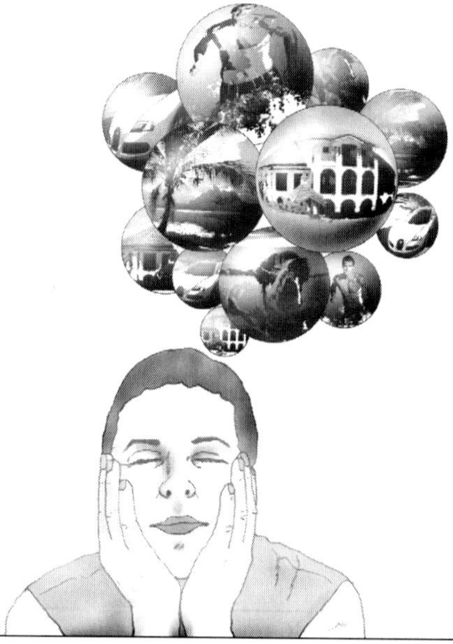

"Dreams are the messages of the soul."

When you wake up, that is, you are half-awake, you are already in the alpha state. You do not need to do deep breathing now because it would probably make you immediately fall asleep again. In the alpha state, you write down – completely uncensored by reason – everything that rises up from within, no matter how seemingly incoherent it may be or stylistically questionable etc. All that is not important now. **What is important is that The Soul writes.** And the next morning, you will be surprised at the realisations that such notes may have on you, which you would have only accessed with difficulty or not at all in your waking consciousness.

Starting soulwriting

Find a current, intense problem for your healing or solution process – as already mentioned, we call it a *project* that you would like to solve. It does not matter whether it is a physical, relationship, work, or financial project. The *KUBYmethod* is in principle equal for all projects.

Collecting pain images: start by writing down everything that hurt or offended you regardless of whether it happened as an adult or as a teen. Now you have the exact project (problem) written down on paper. Not all projects can be solved at once. Get ready to work on your various construction sites one at a time. Otherwise there will only be unfinished buildings in your life, and you will lose the pleasure and the confidence to become happy *and* healthy in a spiritual way with the *KUBY-method* and to remain so.

Also write down the moments in which you were hurt or offended which cannot be changed because the person involved may be unavailable or doesn't want to see you, or may have even died, or something else. Write everything as if it were happening right now, at this moment. **It is absolutely important to always write in the present tense, no matter when the scene or anything similar took place!**

Resurgence of a pain image and its reconstruction: in addition write everything down that was spoken in the scene in direct speech, word for word; that is, not in the third person, but always only in literal speech and in the first person. For example, do not say: He or she said …, but: Dad: " …" Me: " …", Mum: " …" and so on; i.e. pure dialogues together with descriptions of action: *Dad put his hand on my left shoulder*, etc. This is unusual, but essential for the healing process. You will later feel that the only texts that have power and authenticity are the ones written in the here and now. You, therefore, put your words in the I-form into the mouth of the persons involved.

The 3 ***most important***
rules for soulwriting:

1. precise

2. precise **!**

! *3. precise*

Avoid general descriptions in the third person, such as "He behaves strange." This is much too imprecise. Write what the persons literally say and exactly what they are doing. In this way, you as a writer and a reader are directly in the process. Their behaviour is thus not "strange", "repressed" or something else, but the person says something like, "Will you make anything of yourself?", or whatever else. It is best to let the persons involved speak as they spoke at the time – that is, if necessary also in their dialect or native language. There is no doubt about whether what you write is true. Your truth is the only truth. And just as an occurrence happened to you, or is coming to your mind now that you think of it, you write it down without commenting or questioning it.

A specific example for soulwriting

A text written in the present tense demands precision: now it is no longer enough to write: "I had a difficult childhood." In the present the sentence must be something like this: "I am a difficult child." But even this sentence is still not in the present, rather it may include a whole epoch of your life.

So how far does rational, analytic thought have to be broken down for it to be experienced in the Now? You may reply, "I was not difficult, my parents were. They were always fighting." Intuitive work is to ask more specifically, for example: "When did I experience them fighting?" The answer may not be "always" or "often", but perhaps it would be, "For example when my father came home drunk after work." But even with such an answer, this is still not intuition. For intuition it has to be: "I'm in the hallway and hear someone trying to put the key in our front (or apartment) door from outside. I know immediately it is dad and I escape to my room. My mother comes out of the kitchen, dad is in the hallway, and mum asks angrily: 'Why are you so late?'"

I describe this fictitious example to clarify the difference between texts of reason and intuitive texts.

The analytical sentence "I had a difficult childhood" or "I am a difficult child" becomes: "I am standing behind the door in my bedroom, shaking all over. Outside the door, mum screams: 'You're drinking away all our money and I'. I'm afraid dad's going to yell back." – and so on.

Write down everything exactly as you experienced it as a young child. When writing, choose details such as: "Mum wears a floral smock. Dad hangs his thick black jacket on the wardrobe hook" lightning fast. And when reason is now criticising you with thoughts like: "How do you even still know that now? It might have been quite different. You're just imagining it", you take no notice at all of these objections. Write down the scene as a literal dialogue as you can see it in your inner eye and as you can feel it again. Supplement this scene with many important details until an example of your "difficult childhood" is recorded exactly. Then you will have your "pain image".

If you have recognised this "difficult childhood" or "difficult child" as the cause of your present illness or your present problem, with the "pain image" you receive the crucial material with which you can create the new, healthy, and happy reality. Without bringing the pain image to your consciousness no cure can be consciously brought about. Neither you nor any other human have ever been made ill by a "difficult childhood". We can only suffer from real experiences, and one of these real experiences is needed in the here and now. For everything that is in the now can be changed now! However, if we leave the pathogenic experiences in the past or on an analytical-abstract level, they are not in the now and therefore cannot be changed or re-written.

This is my soulwriting *method*®. You write almost intuitively. That is, it is not I who writes, it is IT, the soul. You simply concentrate on the fact. You do not step out of the scene that you have by the coattails. It is about staying with the scene, no matter how fragmented or strange the images appearing inside you may be. All this is part of the intuitive search for the pain image, which comes to light when soulwriting.

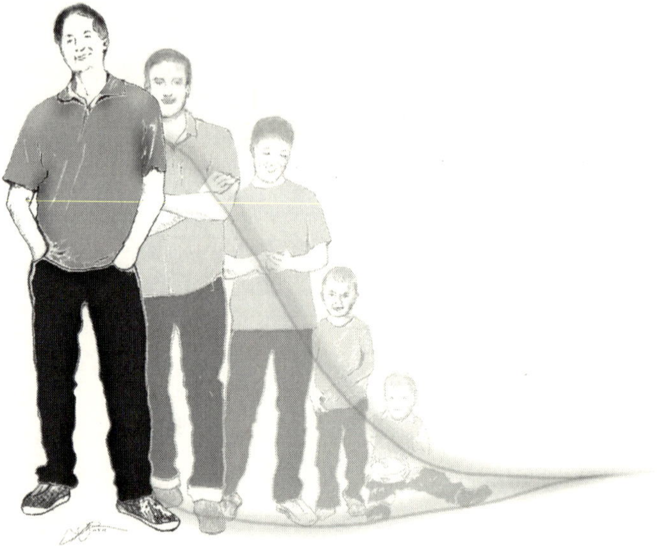

"Every person is connected with their infinite past in many forms."

When writing, no one should disturb you or ask what you are writing. Even if you have someone whom you trust, do not say anything, just write it down. Only after that can you read it out to this person if you have a truly open relationship and they want to help you improve your situation. This gives you the opportunity to not only reflect on your experience alone but also through the eyes of someone else. This is what writing it down is for. Even if there is no one to read your soulwriting to, just reading back your own writing (out loud, if possible) yields insights that would never have come through pure thought or memory.

You can give your soul a voice, lend it your hand and a pen (or the PC keyboard) and let IT write. Since it is not you who is writing, rather you are writing on its behalf, your questions can also be answered immediately. You write your questions exactly the same as the answers – neatly separated, just as the dialogues between the actors are listed in a screenplay. You do not ask your soul to make sense, meaning that you immediately understand what it says. Even if your mind finds that it writes the greatest nonsense – often understanding comes later on when reading it aloud and/or with multiple written inquiries.

You can write this dialogue with your soul for many pages – until everything is clear to you. You only have to be undisturbed and free so that you can express yourself as it comes: laughing, crying, screaming, feeling shame, or anything else. No one can take offence. If it has to be more powerful and you are worried you will be uncomfortable, then scream into a pillow, or go out and scream in the woods or in a meadow, where you can behave as you like. In any case, everything that grieves you should be on paper; even the most amazing, strangest stories that do not seem to have anything to do with your present life; if you see them before your inner eye and even "experience" them again – then put them on paper (or in a file – and do not forget to save it!).

Even if you think that you are making it all up, tell yourself: imagination is the sum of all lives, and thus humans cannot really make anything up. Any story that comes from within you has meaning, you simply have to look at it closely and be careful not to jump from one story to the next. Stay with the one that was shown to you in your project (problem), even if it was only an image in your head.

It is like a puzzle that you put together. But you have no template and no idea what the end result will be. You may see something you cannot classify. Write it down and question it; see what comes next, write it down and question it again.

You need to know what was, what is coming, where you are, who is with you: Are you a man or woman, how old, indoors, outside, winter, summer? You want to know exactly.

You can write a whole novel, but in doing so, always ask yourself, "What does this story have to do with what I suffer from today, in this life? What does it have to do with the project (problem/ symptom) I have chosen for this process?" In this way, you will soon find stories, events, and very precise scenes in this and/or a different life that contain a conflict that is still unresolved, which still causes you problems, worries, grief, and pain. This scene is then what we call in the *KUBYmethod* the already mentioned *pain image*. If you have this image in your consciousness, that is, you can see it clearly before you and know what happened to you or through you, then this is the material for your healing or the solution to your problem. It is transformed by rewriting. See more on the next page.

Changing the pain by writing

When you have found the pain image through soulwriting, you begin healing by "rewriting." This means: you read through all your texts again, and if you can make more details clear, add them to the text. It is therefore of great advantage to copy the handwritten text literally (together with all deficiencies) typing it into the computer (if you have not already used it from the beginning), and add the texts (if necessary with a different type colour). As a result, the self-healing process becomes more and more intense as well as more and more effective. The more precisely the painful scene is recorded in the present and in literal speech, the more thorough the healing can be.

I emphasise it again: *These two styles – literal speech and the present tense – are of paramount importance for how effective rewriting will be! (Intuition does not know time, everything can only be in the now.)*

Rewriting gives the imagination a new reality with which the old painful reality is retrospectively replaced by a healing experience.

Writing down your way to happiness

As accurate and as real as the story of suffering turned out, as real is rewriting it now into a story of happiness. This story, however, does not emerge separately, as if the story of suffering had never existed – no, you let the story of suffering develop until the suffering becomes too much for you.

You do not want to accept suffering anymore: and right at this point, you begin to defend yourself, to give yourself respect, to lock the tormentor away, to make clear to them that they must immediately and instantly cease with their intolerable behaviour. Regardless of the reasons for their painful behaviour (because that is all to be understood – or not), you tell them here and now on paper quite clearly, where their limits are.

If resistance is too powerful, then this is just one more aspect of your story, which you can also rewrite. It should not remain the same as it happened the first time because it makes you ill. Everything that is in your creative power and imagination is used to end this old painful horror for you once and for all.

Changing the attitude of the persons involved: write down what the culprits have to say in their apology. You do have time and understanding, but you have no understanding if they do not change now and immediately. If they cannot, or if this would not serve your reconciliation, you can also exercise revenge and punish them mentally or in writing, as required by your sense of justice. Just keep in mind that you do not want to become a murderer yourself, because that would not make you happy in the long run. Defend yourself in such a way that on the one hand, you can finally express enough on the part of your oppression, your ill-treatment, and your humiliation, and on the other hand, so that you are exhausting your anger completely.

In the end, however, the demon that has tormented you must be pacified. Because even a demon, a criminal, a child molester – everyone has a heart, and at the end of your rewriting this heart must also have found your tormentor. Perhaps it will turn out that they were only "a very poor fellow," but this is no longer an excuse for a brutal, human-contemptuous action.

If you achieve this in your rewriting, this person is ultimately purified from insight and remorse, and invariably asks you forgiveness for all that they have done to you. They vow to change from now on. If they cannot, or if it is too easy for them, then expose them to the scene of social ostracism described by you. Make their crime publicly known in your imagination.

Let everyone see what they did to you. If this is embarrassing to anyone in your environment, the time has now come for everyone to be completely behind you and publicly take your side, which should be written down. Write it all down. It is your healing.

Compacting the new reality: in the end, if you can accept your tormentor's apology because it is genuine, then you have done your healing. Everything you have ever suffered and that led to your problem today is now transformed and pacified. An entirely new relationship has been created with the former culprit, because even this person has a soul, which they finally discovered due to your rewriting.

What is crucial is that you are pushing this process forward. You put the liberating phrases in your mouth when writing about your tormentors; you have them act as you need them to for your happiness. If you do not, nothing changes. This is your healing process; the tormentors will not help you. You test your feelings for what is necessary, so that you are completely liberated from all sorrow, all hurt, all grudges, all hatred, everything that has ever made you angry and miserable, and everything you could never have forgiven.

In the end the purified reality is even humorous. Your new life should be fun. You can be happy, you can be funny, and all the others involved in the scene can be as well. You allow the healing which is created by your imagination to all who have created pain for you. You have freed yourself and them from all evil. There is nothing left to remember about your old destiny, it disappears into laughter at your new, self-created reality. Laughter is the best medicine. Because laughter has a frequency that directly forms synapses which spread different information to the cells that had previously been living in fear and fright, that is to say, a vibration that awakens them to an entirely new life.

If you have completed the rewriting fully, the symptom will say goodbye, because its message has arrived. Peace has been established. Love prevails.

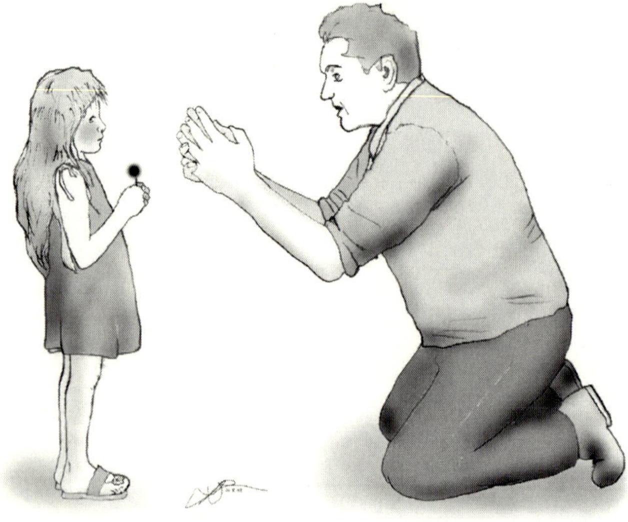

"Even a wrong-doer can ask for forgiveness."

Insofar as the central definition of soulwriting. Here is a general note to pain and reconciliation: understandably reconciliation can also be superficial without knowing exactly what is being reconciled. Because it is certainly not pleasant to look at the crime, the injury, or the misfortune, or whatever it was, again and again. But at the very least, it should be clear what the reconciliation is about. It is hardly a real reconciliation to say, "I forgive you." Reconciliation only happens if a new behaviour is actually shown – a behaviour that includes and expresses reconciliation. This new type of character has a new quality, and this cannot be produced by a fast process.

But even if rewriting is "merely" about an imagined reconciliation, there is no need to discuss this point – the disappearance of the symptom is the proof that the reconciliation has taken hold. Medicine that cannot perceive this process on a spiritual-soulful level calls such cures *spontaneous recovery* (see also "Five Human Images"). But anyone who has gone through this process knows that nothing has been cured spontaneously. In the case of rewriting, a highly concentrated, sometimes even a very exhausting, intensive writing process is required. It can sometimes even go on for days and weeks, until the rewriting has been carried out so specifically and precisely on paper that it includes complete liberation. This is self-healing through self-work. And this makes you competent.

It is also work to even find the pain image before rewriting; to admit and to deal with the emotional agony of reliving it – all this has little to do with spontaneous healing, but very much with an expansion of consciousness, with bringing light into darkness. That purely mental work achieves a physical effect cannot be imagined in materialistic philosophy and is therefore not possible. But once you have successfully gone through the process of soulwriting, you will feel in your own body or soul that only through your spiritual work can breathtaking changes be possible.

The beauty of the *KUBYmethod* is that with our present awareness, we create a harmonious solution for a previous event. Harmony represents the highest consciousness, because harmony can also be translated as love. And where love prevails, we are in harmony with the universe. Who could ask for more?

Overview of the 10 most important factors when soulwriting:

1. Always choose only one problem (project).
2. Write down the problem as specifically and vividly as possible, not in medical terms, but purely emotionally (injuries, illnesses, health, etc.).
3. People who are also involved in this project must also be clearly described.
4. Dialogues not in the third person, but directly, i.e., reproduced in direct speech.
5. Only in the present tense (everything is always happening NOW)!
6. While writing, let all the emerging emotions run free – even with the courage for anger.
7. Do not impose a limit on the soul dialogue, but write until a clear, coherent feeling for the core of the matter arises.
8. Rewrite the pain image, the burdensome situation you find in a new, liberating reality until you have a happy ending.
9. Be able to forgive (yourself and others).
10. Peace and harmony are felt in the healing process that begins with the imagination.

Two self-healing stories

Daniel, 46 years

Since he was 16, Daniel has suffered from *Crohn's disease*[1]. He has already had multiple hospital stays. He now feels so miserable that he has been ill for over a year and cannot live without high doses of cortisone and azathioprine, as his doctors prescribe. He has to go to the toilet almost every hour and therefore can hardly leave his apartment. His bowel movements are usually no more than brown water, which comes out with pressure. Daniel is getting thinner, his circulation is very unstable, and he has little energy.

"All the doctors I've met – and there have been many – cannot offer anything other than chemicals and surgery. I've had it with both of them," he says. "None of what I've been given to me over the last 30 years has made me healthier – on the contrary. I'm always having new symptoms like constant joint pain, immobility in my arms and legs, and I have an inflamed, very painful toe." A naturopath who told him honestly that she could not help him recommended my book *"Healing – the Miracle inside you"* to him.

1 Details and names have been changed in the self-healing stories to protect privacy.

Daniel began to work with the book. He realised that he had to change his human image that he had taken from the doctors to be able to heal himself. For the first time, he did not regard his symptoms as medical, but human. He did not think he had Crohn's disease, but simply had "the shits." Since medicine usually responds to the question of what the cause of Daniel's suffering might be with: "There's nothing to it," or makes vague, biochemical assumptions which do not lead to healing, Daniel himself now began to search for the cause. Like any disease, it was his very personal story, and there was a lot to it for him. My book made him realise that he would only be healthy if he found and healed this personal cause. No one could do it for him.

According to *the KUBYmethod*, the symptom itself points to the cause. For this, the person affected and a medical layman only needs to ask: What is having "the shits" saying to me (in this case)? In other words: what is the message of the symptom? You do not have to speculate or have a high level of knowledge for the answer, but simply look at the facts. The fact is Daniel regularly has diarrhea. What is more obvious than to ask: "When does a person shit their pants?" Every child knows the answer: "when they are afraid."

So did Daniel sense that he knew where the *fear* came from? A lot of inner images emerged for him simply by asking the question. Daniel had suffered from this symptom for decades, but no one had ever pointed out the connection between body and mind, even though it is obvious.

It is *important* when soulwriting with the *KUBYmethod* that the images that come into consciousness are not only seen and thought, but are immediately written down following the rules of the method: in the present tense and in word for word speech. Not descriptively or analytically, but like that:

Daniel writes at night:

We are sitting at the kitchen table in the kitchen at home in Grillparzer Street. The kitchen is small, narrow, and with brown decoration. The tiles are yellow and have a kind of sunflower pattern, they continue around the kitchen table. The table is on the right in the corner so that two people can sit on each side of the long side. I – about 7 years old – sit on the right in the back; behind me is the refrigerator which means I can't get out. Next to me is my sister Anke, two and a half years older. I am opposite my father, my mother is next to him, so she can always jump up.

My father comes to eat lunch from our electric shop out front, like every day. He sits down at the set table. He has never helped my mother. I feel that he is tense. Nobody says anything. I am afraid. The silence is eerie. Suddenly my father says to me, "Why are your fingernails so dirty?" All my intestines pull together jerkily. I suddenly feel ill. I do not dare say anything. My mother answers for me.

Mother: "Leave the boy alone."

Father: "Why are you getting involved?"

My sister says, "Do you always have to be so loud?"

I want to sink into the ground under the table in fear.

Father shouts across the table: "I'm not loud," and throws the cutlery onto his plate. He jumps up and orders my mother: "Let me out of here."

I feel like I'm going to puke, but I cannot get a word out. I just stare in front of me and keep eating, albeit slowly.

Dad runs out of the kitchen, my mother says, "Leave him, he'll calm down soon."

Father: "I heard that" he shouts from outside the door.

We say no more, only our cutlery rattles. I can't really swallow another bite, but keep eating, so I'm not the cause of any more criticism. I'm full of fear. Suddenly father comes back in: "Let me through," he snaps at my mother and sits down. We eat until we're finished without saying another word. I would be the last person to say something. My stomach is as hard as a steel ball, the fear is pounding up to my neck, my father could have a fit of rage at any moment.

Such a scene is called as already stated above a *pain image*. Its transformation from fact to fiction (the *rewriting*) must now be as credible as possible so that neither scepticism nor doubt arise. Self-healing is not magic, as people would like medicines or healers to be, either by a chemical input or an energetic one that you do not have to understand. The *KUBYmethod* requires work, concentration, and discipline. You create a difference from what made you sick and contribute to love in the universe. If Daniel's parents become loving people through his rewriting, his symptom has fulfilled its task and disappears. This rewriting is as follows for Daniel:

My aunt Teta is visiting Grandma who lives downstairs in the house. I stand at the top of the staircase and see her go to Grandma's room. "Teta, I have something to tell you, can you come upstairs?" This almost makes me cry. "Of course, what's going on?" She comes up. I shut the door of my room behind us. We sit. She puts her hand on my shoulder: "You're crying – what is it, my little one?"

Me: I'm so afraid of Dad.

T: But why?

M: He scares me every lunch time. He screams and yells at me.

T: Why?

M: He has a bad temper. I don't know. There's always something he doesn't like.

T: What does mum do?

Me: She just says he should calm down. But that makes him angry, and he runs off.

T: And Anke?

M: He screams at her too, then she keeps quiet.

T: And you?

Me: (I can't hold my tears back anymore): I don't do anything at all. I almost die of fear.

T: Is it like this every lunchtime? She strokes my head and takes me in her arms.

Me: Yes, it's very bad.

T: Then I'll say something. This is unacceptable.

Me: Really? You'll do that?

T: Yes, and you say something too.

Me: I don't dare to.

T: He won't do anything to you. I'll make sure. I'll stand outside and come in at once if he goes for you.

Me: Yes, really?

T: Yes. I'll come up when you're eating. First I'll go down to check on grandma.

I'm excited. Today is my day. Teta is here and will help me – amazing! I'll say something immediately when he begins, I'll do something. I trust myself. I'll tell him everything I think and that I feel that he ruins everything. I go into the kitchen and sit, as always, in my spot. My heart is pounding. It's tingling inside me, I feel fear, but also courage. That is new. Dad comes in, sits down and begins to eat without saying a word. Suddenly he says to me: "Why do you have such dirty fingernails?" What do I do now? Before I say a word, my mother says "Leave the boy alone." Father yells at mum: "Don't get involved".

The door opens, and Aunt Teta comes in the room.

I call out: Teta, Teta!

Anke: Hello, Teta.

Father: What are you doing here? (She is his sister.)

T: I'm visiting grandma and just heard you yelling.

F: I'm not yelling.

Me: Yes you are! You always scream and scare me.

T: Karl-Ernst, you can't scare the boy.

F: I don't scare him.

Me: Yes you do, you always scare me. I almost die of fear. With you, we never know when you're going to scream. We never know why. I always think you're about to beat us all to death.

T: Look the boy in the eyes. Do you really want him to be so afraid of his dad?

F: He doesn't need to be afraid.

Me: Why don't you stop then? I always think I'm to blame for everything. I can't keep thinking that. It's making me sick. I'm already sick. I always have a stomach ache.

T: Do you hear that?

F: (looks at me) Is this true?

Me: (I can't help crying) Yes. I always think you're going to kill us all.

F: I would never do that.

Me: (crying) But you act like you will.

F: No.

A + M (both together): Yes you do!

T: Take a look at this. You're breaking your family.

Dad starts to panic. He feels fenced in: "Let me out."

Mum lets him out immediately.

T: Stay here!

F: Get out of my way!

Aunt Teta does not budge a single inch. I think it's great. She is strong.

T: You'll listen for once!

He tries to avoid her gaze. He stands insecurely in the kitchen.

T: Now sit down and listen.

I sit on my chair and am now quite big. Teta nods at me. Dad sits down.

T: So, Daniel, tell dad again what you told me.

M: (gathering all my courage): If you think I am going to listen to your shouting at lunch every day and sit fearfully in the corner, you're wrong.

Dad freezes. His facial features become hard.

Me: You don't hit me.

T: That would be better!

Me: You make me sick, dad. You make us all sick, can't you see that?

His face trembles.

Me: You are going to be sick too, you destroy me, and all of us including yourself.

Mum has an expression as if thunderstruck, but she does not stop me. I believe she thinks it's right.

Me: Right, Mum?!

Mum nods. Dad sees that. Suddenly he is very small.

A: Daniel is right, I can't stand it.

Father quietly says to mum: Let me out.

She lets him out, and Teta steps aside. He goes out into the hallway.

Fear rises up in me: What is he doing now?

A: (calls after him): Stop! Just stop it!

It gets very quiet outside. Now I am silent too. We are all silent. Suddenly we hear him sobbing outside. We look at each other questioningly. I say to Anke: "Let me out." I go to the door, open it slowly, look carefully around the corner to the left. Dad is, in fact, crouching on the first step of the stairs, head in his hands.

I go to him. Now I'm a head taller than him. I stroke his head and cheek for the first time in my life. (*I feel it. It is not a text. I feel it.*) We say nothing. He takes his right hand from the face and grabs my right leg. I kneel down. His hand comes up. He takes me in his arms and whispers with tears in his voice: "I'm sorry." I have to cry too.

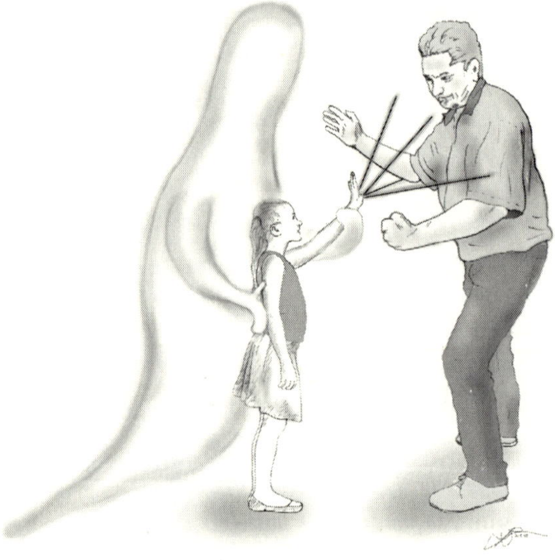

"Those who must defend themselves receive help when they imagine it."

Mum, Anke, and Teta are standing in the doorway. They have tears in their eyes. He feels they are there and stretches his arm out to mum and Anke. They come closer and kneel with us. Dad wraps his arms around all of us and weeps bitterly. We cry too.

He says: "I am so exhausted. The business is too much for me. – I don't want to do it ever again, I don't want to do it ever again, I am so sorry – so sorry." He gives me a kiss, and I sense the salty taste of his tears.

F: It's all so bad because business is bad. I don't have enough work for the staff. All of this makes me so frustrated.

M: It's good that you're saying this to the kids, they always think they're to blame.

F: (looks at mum) But you know how I mean it.

M: Yes, but do you not see the fear in Daniel's eyes?

F: No. (He looks at me questioningly): Really?

M: Always!

Dad takes me in his arms and holds me close.

M: I think you'd rather do something different than the shop.

A + me (almost simultaneously): No? – For real? – But what?

F: I'm running the shop for you all.

M: I don't believe that. You do it because you inherited it from your mother.

F: (to Teta) Because of you I had to take over the shop.

T: Because of me???

F: Because you left home so early, I had to run the business on my own when our father died.

T: You don't have to keep doing it for me if it's making you unhappy, and your children are living in fear and dread – leave it!

Me: What would you do instead?

F: Music, to entertain people, to make people happy – that's my dream job.

M: And I would like to be a teacher again. Let us start again, honey. Let's sell everything and start somewhere else.

A: I would also like to go somewhere else.

I am totally surprised. Suddenly everything is resolved.

F: (hugs us children and asks mum) Will we manage it, starting again from scratch?

M: Yes, definitely, if you do your thing and I do mine, we'll be strong together. We can do everything. The main thing is peace.

F: I won't shout anymore. I don't have to shout anymore. (And then he looks at me and says): Then there is no more fear!

I take a step toward him and wrap my arms around his neck. He holds and hugs me. Weights are falling off my body. I only say: "Oh, lovely!"

This is a small part of Daniel's self-healing process. This is precisely how the pathogenic causative energies of a modern symptom can be described. Since the brain cannot distinguish between fact and fiction, this new experience means that the synapses are no longer created by fear, but by respect, love, and understanding. These are completely different messengers for his digestive track than those of the last 30 years. The beauty of this work is that the new healthy and happy reality creates a vibration that reaches the father.

As Daniel's father was still alive, he called Daniel shortly afterwards and showed personal interest in him for the first time in his life. For Daniel this was a miracle. But it isn't really a miracle because he knew how he had brought about this change of character in his father – even if he did not explain it to him, but of course accepted it gratefully. Thus the father had the feeling that his call had broken the ice. Both were happy about their success, making Daniel's physical health process progress rapidly (inexplicable to medicine). As mentioned, medicine calls this "spontaneous recovery". In reality it was anything but spontaneous. It took intense, highly concentrated work for Daniel to create this new reality for himself.

Many attendees of my seminars experience similar events in one form or another. People whose unsuccessful treatment had cost them over 100,000 USD over the years were now curing themselves for only a few hundred USD. A success rate and cost savings that to date only one Swiss health insurance (*EGK* Gesundheitskasse) has recognised and therefore covers my seminars for their members.

Numerous examples can be cited: the University of Ulm (Germany), for example, would have an appraisal (or study) on the actual success rate of the *KUBYmethod* if it were to be commissioned by a health insurance company. I myself would welcome such scientific, neutral expertise, because in general people find it very difficult to explain these purely spiritual healing processes. It can only be understood if you have experienced such a cure with your own body.

Ines, 47 years old

Here is the example of Ines, who has suffered from a bad back for years. Finally operating could no longer be avoided because between the 4th and 5th lumbar vertebrae the intervertebral disc was displaced by half an inch, as the CT clearly showed. On the Friday before the operation, Ines called me and was regretful that she had only just heard of me and my method, but next Tuesday she would be operated on by a really excellent doctor, which she was very happy about. She only wanted to know from me if it would still make sense to go ahead with the *KUBYmethod* in spite of the operation to find out the cause of her back pain. Of course it makes sense, since as long as the cause is not fixed, the surgery can only have an effect on the symptom, but not cure it. Healing requires a life change depending on the cause.

On Monday, Ines called again and reported that the hospital had postponed the surgery until Thursday for internal reasons. She did not have to admit herself until Wednesday afternoon. She wanted to know if I had time prior to this to work with her. I took the time and assisted her over one and a half hours with her self-healing process, something I do with many seminar attendees on the weekend. But because of the date of her surgery, she could not wait until then.

I recorded the conversation with Ines (for self-protection) so that nobody could claim that I talked her out of the surgery. The next day the surgeon made an X-ray of her back for safety, and saw that Ines' intervertebral disc had receded by half. She told him that she "had rewritten" the cause of her symptom. The surgeon said that he did not understand anything about that, but since it had been so successful she should definitely continue with it, and he could no longer justify an operation in this case.

Ines now has an entirely healthy back. The rewritten cause was a move at the age of 13, which her father had imposed on the family. For Ines, this meant: away from her roots, her friends, and her first bashful love. In the half-hour of "rewriting," she (as a 13-year-old) enforced her interests over her idolised and beloved father's (a captain in the navy) for the first time, for her mother had never been able to do so either. For Ines, it was a real event, accompanied by many tears and a lot of shouting, which she authentically experienced until her highly authoritarian father relented.

A script for the new reality

The basis for your new (as happy and healthy as possible) reality is the "script". This is how you create your goal. Write down the "movie" that you want to live out. This gives your actions a new direction. In other words, the actions receive a new matrix or pattern, a new vibration. To create this quality of experience is human creativity, from which freedom, competence, and self-determination emerge. They can no longer be driven through life, but create themselves. All this always begins in the mind.

Here is an example: Take any random scene, preferably a current one that you still fully remember or perhaps is even in progress. Record it exactly in the word for word sequence as it happened (or is happening). Then look for the moment in your text where you would like to react differently if you could react. On paper you can impose such behaviour on yourself and others that is far from what happened in reality. Consider the props and actions that might help your new reality, such as a bouquet of flowers, or going to the movies, or incense, or a very dimmed light. Imagine your role and those of your fellow actors in this new atmosphere. Exactly like you already know from *soulwriting*, write exactly what words, actions, and movements are necessary to make your intention come to the fore.

With these texts (scripts) you build, so to speak, an intermediate stage between the present and the desired future being.

Without this intermediate stage this new being usually does not emerge. On paper a matrix, so to speak, emerges for a new healthy and happy life.

Neurobiology and brain research can perfectly prove that our brain is there to create our own reality. Normally – as we have been taught to date – we were of the opinion that reality exists independently from the brain. The brain uses our five senses to perceive reality and is not there to create it.

However the new, still untrained concept means that since our diseases and our health are clearly part of our reality, we also create our diseases and our health with our brains. A shocking idea that neurobiology conveys to us. You might get the idea that this means people are responsible for their own diseases. But this is not a nice and, above all, not a helpful idea. Because diseases are never about guilt, but always about development.

If we pay even more attention to what brain researchers tell us, then their thesis – or is it really a realisation? – seems to be correct. If we measure brain activity during a perception with an EEG (electroencephalogram), we can say that the centres for the sense organs – sight, hearing, touch, feel, and taste – are only involved in a maximum of 9%! That means over 90% of brain activity is occupied with itself when perceiving reality. Understanding what you perceive by seeing, hearing, smelling, and so on, is thus created in your brain. Your sense organs are merely used to confirm what you want to perceive. Thus there can be no objective perception, as some worldviews would hold. Everything is a matter of interpretation, as emphasised in this book multiple times. You will be dealing with this realisation and its challenges – as you will notice – all your life, especially in terms of health.

Make it clear to yourself that if the five senses are less than 10% involved in perception, there can certainly be no objective truth. If over 90 per cent of all perceptions is caused by prejudices, beliefs, habits, etc., anything that a person describes as truth can only be about their own subjective truth, never a supposedly objective, valid-for-all truth.

If this is the case, make something of it! The more your consciousness expands to a spiritual image, the more the contents with which you "feed" your consciousness will change. Positively thought up and imagined realities uniquely reflect your own creativity, with which you will align and determine your life in joy and confidence. In my seminars I always experience how astonishing and electrifying it is to see how every expansion of consciousness is immediately visible externally. This is not only my impression, but that of the whole group and the camera, if the process is being filmed. Multi-day seminars often act as a "beauty miracle", which attendees often refer to outside the seminar.

To those who make spirit
the boss of their life a new world
will open up.

With the *KUBYmethod*, as we have already seen, rehabilitation or problem solving is always connected with an expanding consciousness. Each step of consciousness makes you not only perceive others differently, but above all yourself as well. By expanding your consciousness, not only does the disease go away, but opportunities for your own future expand as well. We increasingly recognise our potential. This is the true meaning of a disease which requires this expansion of consciousness for healing to occur.

Even if life is often challenging and tests you, always remember that you can be the creator of what is to change. In this way, you will feel less like a victim, and instead you will recognise your own greatness, which you must courageously accept – for yourself and for the benefit of everyone. Simply start writing your screenplay and become the director of your life!

4

Self-love is the beginning of all love

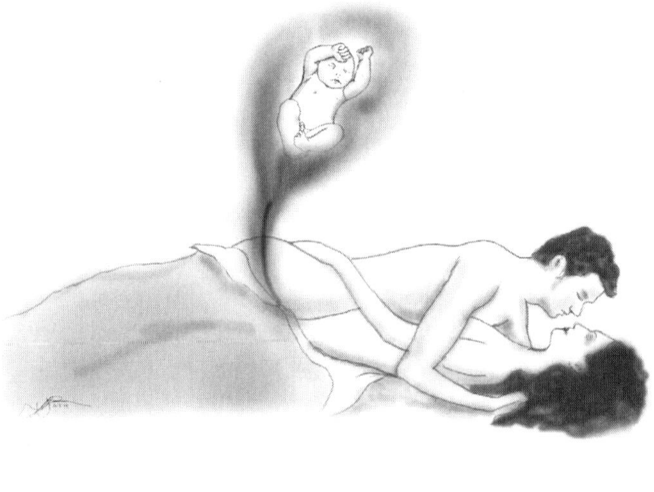

"This decision to incarnate now or later is the most important one in your whole life."

Compassion begins with feeling

If you carry within yourself a human image that does not cling to any matter and recognises everything that exists as a consequence of spiritual impulses, you are no longer following dogma, but your own impulses. Spiritual impulses cannot be absolutised unless they are explained as the only valid truth, as many religions do. With an inner distance, this absolutisation can also be seen as a spiritual impulse. Since you are now a little more familiar with the KUBYmethod and have perhaps even gained practical experience, you know that your mind is free and can imagine anything you want. If it wants to imagine something as the absolute truth, this is a virtual, self-created, or accepted concept – nothing more.

I have already explained in detail in this book that truth can no longer be disputed – it does not exist objectively, it is anchored only in the subjective. This philosophy can lead to real tolerance. You will experience how liberating and fulfilling this is! Interest for your fellow humans grows. You try to understand out of curiosity: what does this woman, this man, or this child consider their truth? Everyone has their own truth, and it is only justified, compassionately, and also necessary, to look closely to find and understand the truth of the other being. But this truth will impress itself deeply within your own inner being and determine further thinking and behaviour.

With this attitude you can also approach animals and have wonderful experiences in communication with them. An animal immediately senses whether you have grasped its truth. So first figure out **who you are for the animal**. You can tell an animal as little as you can a human about whether the image that exists in their head over the other is true or not. This subjective image is always true, because it is the image with which you appear to this animal, and this is where your communication starts.

If you realise that your subjective brain works like this, then you can modulate your image from the other side. You do not need to think "Oh, what a cute little dog", but if you look closely, you might think, "Oh, what a great personality!" and behave accordingly. And already the animal changes the image it has of you in the first moment due to its experience with such beings. If you have some patience and a lot of sensitivity, you can also experience this with animals that are timid with humans.

In this way, you will not only get in touch with yourself, but also with others – whether human or animal. You should not demand anything, neither from yourself nor from others. Only concern yourself with what is. Once you expend energy to achieve something, your compassion will starve. Even if you are asked by others to help them with their healing, you have no other task than to **be present with a completely open heart**. Because if you really want to help, then you only have to be interested in the person's soul. With this attitude compassion emerges on its own.

Compassion is simply overflowing energy without intention. For every healing, it is only about the being knowing itself for whom you feel compassion. You, therefore, have no right to tell him what to do or not to be healthy and happy. This would be ego-controlled, overbearing, alien, and has nothing to do with compassion; even if you are a thousand times right in that your insight, your wisdom, your suggestion would make these people healthy and happy. Others are just as divine as you. But if you can reflect it for them, you are really helping them. You are then automatically loving, friendly, and compassionate.

You do not have to be enlightened to be compassionate. It is better to be compassionate before you are enlightened, because otherwise, enlightenment becomes an ego trip. Compassion is the direct path to losing your ego. You have freed yourself from suffering, even great suffering. However, your joy in your happiness will be lucky only if you can see how someone with whom you have contact also frees themselves from their suffering. When there are more and more who free themselves from their suffering, **this will bring great joy** where everyone has fun. You simply love everyone, because everyone has a soul. And their soul is reflected in yours. There is no situation where this would not be possible.

Unless you are in discord with your own soul. You struggle with yourself and put yourself down so that you can only yell and scream: "Why is no one helping *me*?" Are they all against me? Everyone only thinks about themselves, no one thinks about me, what immeasurable injustice." And so on.

Where and how did you lose your self-love? Perhaps you are living your daily life in constant overload and no longer know whether you are coming or going. Perhaps too much responsibility has been inflicted on you, and you keep your feelings under control so as not to collapse. Perhaps it was and still is disappointing experiences that have always set back your self-esteem.

If this is the case, please correct this course right away! Begin by having a little dialogue with yourself – you will always be able to manage a few minutes a day. Consciously treat yourself to something in the meantime: building thoughts, a good cup of tea, your favourite flowers, a song you haven't heard in a long time, a little walk. Listen to the birds chirping, put your face in the sunshine, or enjoy the refreshing rain. It is the little treasures of everyday life that give life more feeling: for yourself and thus for others, for life in general.

Regardless of whether you are dealing with yourself or another person, real help happens only through compassion. And this requires true self-love. In any case and of course in this sort of case, you can only help if you have compassion. For this, you must be completely fearless. However, if you are afraid of the suffering that you reflect to others, then you sincerely say, "I'm sorry, I cannot help you." If the fear is transferred, there is a danger that inner distance occurs. We want to protect ourselves through distance because we feel overwhelmed meeting every being lovingly. But is it not the case that we argue more often with people whom we particularly love (for example, a spouse, mother, father, children)? It should, therefore, be possible to love people and other beings with whom we never argue.

Try it: With every person you meet, even complete strangers who you only see briefly, think: "I love you." You will be amazed how easy it is to create a loving environment.

If you cannot have this loving thought with each person, then you should briefly look at the people with whom you often argue, but with whom you are ultimately connected by love. After this, you can also inwardly say to the person with whom you are dealing in a good or less good way: "I love you!" You will find after a while that this sentence works wonders. It also affects the people with whom you are very closely connected.

Repeat this phrase internally as often as you can: "I love you. I love you. I love you. I love you. I love you …" And you will be surprised again.

With this love, which is also self-love, love for God, or love for this universe in addition to love for Mother Earth and Father Sun, we can conclude peace with all relationships and the conflicts contained therein. With voluminous self-love, we can always give, even to our hitherto most harsh enemies, adversaries, enviers, pessimists, naggers, sufferers, lamenters, poor souls, the injured, distressed, cheaters, rulers, tormentors, scoundrels – whatever creature: with self-love we can encounter everyone better than with self-doubt, self-hatred, self-denial, self-reproach, or self-insecurity.

Either you are part of the problem
or you are part of the solution.
You have to choose.

With self-love, you can "afford" to have compassion. In fact, you will not want it any other way, and you will not be able to do otherwise. Through compassion, you can look at everything around you differently: with respect, mindfulness, and truthfulness for what it is. Compassion gives everyone freedom and remains in good connection with it. And that alone leads to more freedom in your thoughts and feelings. **Compassion is based on self-love**, which is free of selfish aspirations and desires. You feel a part of the great whole, as part of the Great Spirit.

Self-love is the only thing you can take with you when all connections tear. Those who can give love will experience love everywhere in this universe. This universe is dedicated to the principle of harmony and the prevention of stress. Even if your habitual way of life is lacking, you will experience love when you have love. Love is a spiritual value; it does not need form. Love can become a form, but it is retained even when the form dissolves or does not occur in the usual way.

So let us produce, accumulate, renew **love** every day through soul hygiene, that is, conflict resolution for yourself and with others. All this has to take place in our minds so that we know how to behave properly and with a smile. Those who love themselves do not bind themselves to concepts. Less is more. When we perceive ourselves as spiritual beings, form is a transitory phenomenon of the mind.

Everything is fine just as it is

All love, as described above, begins with self-love, so you reestablish where your world was still in order. Ultimately, where your body created it. What skills did you have then? What fascinated you as a child? That's where you connect.

It is never too late to begin with what was actually planned during your procreation. Your soul always has a life plan that works for the benefit of all. The soul has nothing to do with selfishness, because everything that can be created with it must be left behind as soon as you change your form. Your life plan does not need spectacular tasks, it can simply consist of serving the heart and, for example, taking responsibility for clean toilets or streets. Pure ego constructs and projects which are mostly at the service money, power, and pride, cost unnecessary effort and are completely in contradiction to the soul's need to be free of stress.

The right life plan does not involve stress, it can also become dramatic, but it is always designed to be in harmony with the world. In order to achieve this, this principle applies: minimum effort, maximum effect. However, implementation is not easy because life consists of many ups and downs. Those who are too far away from their life plan and are waiting too long to react to changing conditions lose their ability to act and his life is dominated by others. This is when accidents, illnesses, and other misfortunes occur, which bring down the current, allegedly correct concept. The way out of this dilemma is again – how could it be otherwise? – by expanding your consciousness. In order to exceed a limit of consciousness, the intention must be formulated, namely, a very specific, precise intention. This allows us to push into new territory which we have not even known to exist or even could exist. If, according to our philosophy, we were to wait for great social discretion, it would be bad for our health.

We can start expanding our consciousness directly here and now. This does more for the global process than theoretical utopias, because good can only be created by good people. Self-healing means taking illness as an invitation to become a better person.

Opening yourself up makes you strong: when we understand ourselves as spiritual beings, we talk about our physical aches, ailments, indispositions, illnesses, and catastrophes not like we usually do, but about which subject the symptom mirrors. Such an approach directs the interest to the person rather than to their environment and adverse circumstances.

This psychological way of looking at something reveals something about the personal conflicts that someone is going through. This is something very private, for which people usually feel ashamed to disclose. Because these personal conflicts may also reveal a weakness. All of us have therefore quickly learnt to blame external factors for our symptoms, because this means we do not have to expose what or who has aggravated, disappointed, or overwhelmed us, and so on. With physical symptoms, we always have an impersonal subject, even if we are bearing the symptoms ourselves: "Oh you poor thing, always catching it!" Or, "If you had dressed warm enough, you would not have a cold now," etc. – people see all of this as better than personal openness and closer scrutiny.

However, as soon as we talk about the mental cause of a disease, our attitude is evaluated. Often we feel unaffected, abandoned, unloved and patronised. Sometimes by our partner, if they are unfamiliar with mentally treating the symptoms. These are all reasons why we would prefer to look at our disease as a result of external conditions and to dispel its true, original causes.

When this happens, you have not only hidden the reasons, but also your soul – and that has to be rejected. The soul is – as already mentioned – only trying to establish harmony. Why, then, should it be hiding and suppressing itself? **Those who do not listen to their soul must feel it**. Those who do not listen to their inner voice may hear it only when their organs begin to complain loudly. If the pain is then removed symptomatically and its cause is not looked at, the soul has no choice but to let the body speak even louder. What other options would it have if its subtle signs are overlooked? It is more difficult to "overhear" pain than the inner voice.

MEN ONLY

"We do not show weakness."

Power, control, competition

A man, a "real" man. What do we expect from him? To be strong, clearly positioned, ready for any delicate situation; a being who is fearless about their existence, who does not shy away from an external argument, and bravely struggles in battle – with armour and visor. In the meantime, he can also arrange a romantic date, take out the rubbish, cook, be there for the birth of your baby, shed tears – but please do it without losing the stony image of "being a whole man".

And the man himself? How do we feel in the face of such stereotypical expectations, which, in spite of opposing assurances of an enlightened, modern-minded society, are still haunting us in our heads?

It is a real burden to fulfil all this. A man is trying to control what he wants to keep in control: in mind, in feeling, in strategies, in action of every kind. Because everywhere a power struggle lurks, and not only in sport. Rivals never rest – neither professionally nor privately: colleagues, business partners, wife or girlfriend, children and neighbours, and finally friends: who is better, who has more, who can do more, who is further ahead? Whoever is ahead has power. You cannot admit weakness (or even show it). No one honours this. So if you do not really feel that well, you downplay it, tell no one, and pretend everything is fine. This attitude costs strength – a lot of strength and makes your inner fire burn out. Burn out is the new disease that many people are proud of, and men especially. Because it has high status in society. After all, you only get burn out if you have been working hard. As a result, everyone knows immediately: He was better than everyone else … But it does not make the person in question happy. He no longer takes any pleasure in this power game, in the competition skirmish, and in putting on a good face for the bad game. Burn – out – out – out – out … Full stop.

And how is it with you? By now, the time has come when you can question your masculine behavioural pattern in order to find out what a so-called weakness really is?

- Do you feel weak if you do not have the solution right away to any situation?
- Do you feel weak when you are worried about someone and show it?
- Do you feel weak when you are worried about your job or about your health?
- Do you feel weak when you feel grief?
- Do you feel weak when you look after your baby?
- Do you feel weak when you spend your free time with your family?
- Do you feel weak when you love yourself – just like that? If you do something that makes sense only to you, something that is more important than anything else?

It is best to put your answers in writing. This means you have them at your disposal if you need an input to think differently in the midst of your consciousness process.

As soon as you have approached the alleged weakness differently, you will find: weakness is recovery, weakness is self-love, weakness is compassion, weakness is life. There is still effort – but not without the soul in the boat. The soul is the helmsman and clock, the ego rows, but only for as long as the soul considers it good and correct, then it takes a break.

Tell yourself in such moments: *Let the others row with their ego in the command post so I do not have to compare myself anymore. My existential angst melts away in the sun of my self-love like ice. Yes, I am weak. Facing the beauty of a relaxed life, I become weak. I do not need anything because I AM. I am weak and free. My emotional and spiritual satisfaction is my most precious asset, which is now competing with nothing and no one. It is as it is.*

This book is a guide to thinking differently. Weakness, in fact, requires a different way of thinking. Health is therefore not a medical issue, but a philosophical issue. And the most delicate thing for men is: *Can I be weak as a man (or can my husband be)? Can it have a high value? Can I stay healthy, happy, and joyful if I am weak?* YES! Because whoever is weak is strong. And above all through the courage to be sensitive. Those who are sensitive are adaptable. Even in evolution, not the strong, but the adaptable have won the race. Those who can adapt must be able to feel. And those who feel also perceive alarm signals if they are under too much stress.

The soul does not want stress, it wants harmony. Because harmony saves energy. Everything that works harmoniously runs almost by itself. Power, control, and competition are then completely superfluous. Perhaps you can take such a new view on the so-called weakness which suddenly shows completely different facets. And if the ego perhaps shuts up in the meantime and you listen to your mental clock more often, you will experience a new lightness.

Look forward to this other kind of power. And whistle happily when someone passes you. Because then, competition is only a game that does not know defeat. And as a change from the dictum, your motto might now be: "Showing weakness is man's first duty." :)

Try it: If you do not have any symptoms or if you can resolve your symptoms relatively quickly and without lasting consequences, you are obviously doing something right. However, if you do not feel full strength, the question is: What do you learn from stagnation, stress, or the feeling of being alone? Each of these points is clear when you have learnt at an intuitive level to communicate with your soul. This is also the *KUBYmethod,* this is also self-healing.

Self-healing is a gate through which you have to step. The more naturally you walk through the gate, the easier it is to get through. Do not hate what is in front of the gate, and do not have any expectations of what comes after the gate. Simply pass through the gate. Because expectation creates fear, anxiety generates expectation – a vicious circle. The passage through the gate happens through written conversation with your soul. The soul includes everything that was, could ever have been, and will ever be or should ever be. Contact with your soul is contact to eternity – it is peace through balance. To arrive there is to accept what is, and serenity in dealing with it is a precious good.

Satisfaction requires mental discipline. Old systems of thought do not dissolve on their own. They must be recognised and corrected every minute by giving them no place. The discipline of serenity says, for example, that what annoys me is not meant to – at least not as my old thinking system would like to interpret it. Even if I do not immediately know how to interpret the event positively – then I interpret it but not in such a way that I would be annoyed. I leave it at first, and as soon as I have a few quiet seconds or minutes to think about it, I seek an interpretation of the event which is supported by peace, health, happiness, and harmony.

If the old thought system can no longer be upset as it is used to, it soon becomes listless and gives up. However, we often still have to bring out the big guns to maintain life. And already we are annoyed, become sick, or lament: "Oh, the world is sooo bad!" Or we attack the people we blame.

The new way of thinking, on the other hand, is based, among other things, on the fact that our brain does not distinguish between reality and illusion. It does not matter if we interpret something as true or untrue, because **truth is also only an interpretation**. And every interpretation produces a feeling that forms synapses in our brain. These, in turn, send messengers that regulate our entire physical system. If we want our physical system to receive only positive, constructive, and healthy messengers, let us allow ourselves only such thoughts (illusions, interpretations of events) that also form such synapses. And this is independent of how other people interpret the same events and see them as true or untrue.

The ability of our brain to control our bodies through synapse formation as we like is almost the last remnant of divinity that we carry within us. Because it is so important, let it be stressed again: **We are the creator of our reality** – exactly what God, the Creator, represents.

WOMEN ONLY

"Can I allow myself that?"

Guilty feelings, lack of self-esteem

At last she made a decision. At last she sees new possibilities, a light on the horizon. But before action is taken – sometimes even in the midst of galloping – suddenly the quiet but stubborn inner voice pops up: "Can I allow myself this?"

Many women are familiar with this feeling: they have freed themselves after some back and forth, look forward to their newly chosen (life's) course – and remain at a standstill or have at least put the brakes on. What is behind this? Often it is her battered self-esteem that is perhaps not yet stable enough, which simply needs a little practice in order to accompany their new life feeling reliably. Frequently it is also personal obligations that seem insurmountable: for example, being there for the ageing parents who need help, for the children who are not yet independent, for their partner, who assumes his wife will keep taking care of everything so he can have his career, for the association, the honorary office where she seems indispensable – and so on and so forth: "You'll manage …"

Of course the fact that others can rely on you is a wonderful, welcoming virtue in human coexistence. Still the whole thing becomes questionable when a woman not only meets her obligations, but lets them take over; when she subordinates herself to her tasks so much that she no longer sees the possibility of finding her personal freedom again.

Where excessive responsibility is borne, there is also the risk of immediate guilty feelings as soon as something goes wrong. Why? At this point, let us ignore the fact that disaster was perhaps already taking place on a sunny day in a pretty orchard when an apple from the tribe of sin was picked. Such hypotheses are not likely to benefit the women of today. Yet many women still feel guilty (much more than men!): "If I had taken better care, then …" "Actually, I should not have said that so directly." "If I had stayed at home, perhaps …" and so on. A woman can spend hours worrying about what she should or could have done. And she soon feels guilty if harmony is disturbed.

A deeply anchored feeling of guilt, which is always associated with a lack of self-esteem, can be distorted in such a way that some women feel guilty even for events of great suffering such as child abuse or domestic violence that were inflicted upon them. They were driven into a situation that left them no way out, and then directed their feelings towards themselves ("Something must be wrong with me …"). What remains is, among other things, a sense of guilt and the secret conviction that "I'm not worth it."

Consequently they are often also reluctant to claim something from life and to take a large piece of the cake. If you feel that you are taking a step backwards in everyday situations or in small or big life decisions too quickly and prefer to let others progress, then make it clear to yourself that in the beginning all you need to do is take a small, but important step: *pause* for a moment! Stop and take in what is happening in your internal resistance; listen, weigh it up, and come to your own centre.

Over time you will come to feel compassion for yourself – for what has been suffered due to injustice and violation. What was, is also NOW. But the now can always be changed as you have learnt from *soulwriting*. Do not hesitate to grab this chance!

And above all: Give yourself the most valuable thing you give to others: *love*. With love, with self-love, you strengthen your self-worth. Love will encourage you to demand something of life, and to take it, quite naturally and without guilt. You can and should allow yourself this gift! With self-love you keep the balance between closeness and boundaries, between obligations and freedom. When you open yourself up to this, you will recognise that you are – without further ado – unique and worthy of love.

Healthy without Medicine: The hardest thing about new thinking is, as you see, to interpret yourself in a positive way. By this I do not mean boasting about yourself, but being free from guilt. You do not have to be perfect. It is simply a question of how to interpret your faults. The subject of guilt is one of the most important factors in self-healing processes because it is often deeply hidden in the subconscious.

If we find, despite intensive investigation of the causes, that there is still resistance to looking at the pain image, the reason (conscious or unconscious) may be guilty feelings in many facets. The cause of a disease or a painful problem is always, as already mentioned, due to ignoring your own soul – either as a victim or as a perpetrator. We often feel guilty about this abuse, even if our own soul has been abused by others and thus great suffering has been inflicted upon us. This often goes so far that sometimes we feel guilty for being born. Some of us have survived an abortion attempt and live with the sense of guilt that we would not exist if it had been up to the will of our mother or others involved.

For some even though they were wanted, they were born as the wrong sex, so to speak. Because the father or mother or both would have so much rather had a boy or a girl, but now this wish is not fulfilled. Those in question already feel guilty in their own skin and often even try to act like the other sex or at least dress themselves to look that way. However since all these attitudes are doomed to failure, the corresponding guilt is carried around with them, though mostly unconsciously. Many feel guilty because their beloved mother was sick and as a child, they felt completely helpless. In addition children can grow up with a great sense of guilt, for example because their father was regularly drowning his sorrow in alcohol. No child would want to accuse their beloved parents of anything – and certainly not of crimes such as rape, sexual abuse, or violence. Before a child takes a stand against their father or mother because of the pain they are suffering, they are more likely to blame themselves and try to do their part to bring peace to the family. The child is ready to bear the blame for everything that is wrong with the family. This is what makes us sick. In order to resolve and cure this disease, the sense of guilt must be dealt with.

In principle the same applies to the perpetrators. Their healing is also blocked by feelings of guilt. It is often even more difficult to resolve because it is easier for the victim to forgive the perpetrator than to forgive yourself as the perpetrator. But this, too, can be achieved with *soulwriting.*

No matter what the cause of a disease or a distressing situation, stress is the overriding and destructive energy. It is the cause of all disease. The soul, however, shows us the way to harmonise every situation, including stress that existed before, the stress that exists at the moment and the stress that is not supposed to exist in the future. As you have seen in this book several times, it is not only necessary to think differently, but to express your change of perspective.

All phenomena can be viewed from an infinite number of perspectives. And each perspective creates a different feeling. A phenomenon from the bird's eye or from the ants perspective, from the biochemical or from the spiritual outlook, etc. – they all come to completely different assessments for one and the same phenomenon. Everyone is right from their own perspective, that is everyone represents their truth.

The most important task is therefore to find and represent your own perspective that best and most directly benefits your own health, love, and harmony – for the benefit of all. This is a task independent of time and place. It also works retrospectively, which is essential not only for the recovery of the individual but for society as a whole, because it is particularly affected by retrospectively-fixed assessments, perspectives, and judgements which burden, create guilt, annoy, insult, offend, or even kill the affected persons.

To change these perspectives, to reevaluate them, to attribute a different, positive outcome to the phenomenon in order to retrospectively produce happiness, love, harmony and being stress free as well as everything that is healthy for yourself and all involved persons – **this is the healing task.**

Humour is ideal for such a change of perspective and for all healing! If we learn not to take our current thought system too seriously, that is, to not make it absolute, then we realise the vital function of humour. Without humour there is no love, without humour there is no health, without humour, there is no joy for life. Martin Luther said, "If God does not understand fun, I do not want to go to heaven." Humour is to question everything and to love everything and everyone – even that what you judge. **Humour is transformation.**

However, humour at the expense of others is not humour, because not everyone can laugh with you. Instead, it is an attack disguised as humour. The attackers are then looking for a counterattack – and the war continues, only by other means. Real humour however should help to resolve the anger, the war, the guilt, the injuries and illnesses and make people healthy. Laughter makes you healthy when it does not make others sick.

The most important and most beautiful humour is to relativise our thought system, that is to show that every phenomenon can also be seen from a perspective that may lead to a significantly different outcome than the usual one. Any perspective in itself may be true. This sort of thought extension is fun and helps to accept the thought system as less absolute. Thus a peaceful, healthy and loving perspective can be exercised, and the corresponding conditions can be put into practise, even where the thought system leads to massive suffering.

And what will you do now with all the suggestions this book has given you so far? The time in which we live brings many challenges for all of us. Both globally and individually. But global changes are always a reflection of the individual. It is therefore a good idea to look after your own personal development. So I ask you: What is the reason you want to expand your potential?

- To gain a higher consciousness?
- To give others greater awareness?
- To connect with the consciousness of many?

Whatever you choose, find your purpose in life. Find something that makes you feel valuable to others – even if it is the frogs you save from the road. The more it is required of you to be helpful and the more valuable and happy it is for the recipient, the more it helps you to develop further. It is also clear that we are able to discover a lot of common ground in human-to-human interaction and this can lift us up. Our sense of security grows with the realisation that ultimately everyone wants to develop and this is subjectively difficult for everyone, no matter where they are in life right now.

If you want to be healthy without medicine, you cannot

achieve this without thinking differently. I hope this book makes this sufficiently clear. Thinking differently changes consciousness. And all big life questions have to do with the development of consciousness. The material level follows from this. **New thinking** begins with what you think about yourself. If it is possible to interpret yourself so that you do not know or see any hostility, then there is no longer any hostility.

When we accept life in all its beauty and dignity, and accept suffering for what it is, we return to peace and confidence. We find a source of primordial energy, from which we can draw a good, fulfilling life. The resulting harmony can be described as love. We are a universe of love. Since the universe is always a spirit in origin, we can also say: **It is the spirit of love from which everything arises.**

The soul does not allow that anyone or anything makes it become corrupt. The soul wants everything, the total harmony we call LOVE.

Appendix

How does Soul Writing work exactly?

Choose how you want to write:

- on your laptop
- with your cell phone
- by hand – in this case note the following:
  - Leave 1⁄3 of the right side of the page blank.
  - Use bound paper. Number the pages.
  - Transfer the text on your computer or on the clemenskuby.com website to the portal "Soul Writing" if you would like feedback from the *KUBYteam*.

1. Write your name, date of birth and your present location on the **first line**.

2. On the **second line** write your **project, in other words** what it is you want to heal or the problem that you'd like to solve. Phrase it as concretely as possible in one or two sentences without using any medical or psychological terms; write down how you experience the restriction of the quality of your life at the moment. The project is the basis for the expansion of consciousness you want to achieve and to which you can always return if you get stuck during your soul writing.

3. Write the current **trigger** on the third line. On what occasion did you last experience this pain or this problem? Was it today, was it yesterday? When was it especially strong (approx. date)? What do you think, could it appear again?

4. Ask yourself: how long have you had the feeling that arose from your project? Follow this feeling and circle around it with questions such as: How old am I when I feel this? Where was it? In what country? What place? Outside or inside? An apartment or a house? In which room? Is it day or night? As soon as you sense even a trace of a concrete event, trust yourself to go deeper into the event. You have to know that it can never become as painful as it has been. Your soul will always open up exactly as much as you can handle, because your soul loves you. The scene which now appears is what the *KUBYmethod* refers to as the **pain image**.

5. **As soon as you have a concrete moment** in sight, you write only in the present tense. From now on there is only the NOW and from this point on you write the scene in the table (see below).

6. In the **first column** (*No.*) the lines are numbered. (The numbering is done automatically on the *KUBYportal.*)

7. In the **second column** (*Person*) you write the name of the person who is currently saying or doing something. The line changes with the person. In a dialogue you also have to change lines if a person only says *"Yes!"* or *"No!"*. In this method of *soul writing*, there is no statement that cannot be assigned to the perception of a specific person. This means that when you write "Me" in the second column, the third column shouldn't be *"The street is narrow"*, but instead *"I am on a wet and narrow street."* In other words, you describe the atmosphere from the point of view of a person and not in a neutral or objective way.

8. When a person appears again, an abbreviation in the **second column** is enough. For yourself you can write ME, for Mom M, for Dad/Father D or F, for Uncle John UJ and so on.

9. What this person is currently saying or doing is written in the **third column** (*Text*) **word-for-word in direct speech**. When something is said, write it down in the authentic original language or dialect if possible.

   a) When writing down this scene from the past, take care to make the **link** to the project clear. This means there is a definite connection between what is currently causing you to suffer and the distress you experience in the scene. You often only become aware of this when you reread the soul writing at a later point in time. You'll discover that you expressed the project or the trigger using the same or very similar words as now appear in the scene.

b) As soon as you are emotionally affected by what is happening in the scene, you've scored a hit. This means that you have arrived at the subjective truth which has to do with your project. This is the scene we call the "pain image".

c) Discipline yourself to such an extent that you write the pain image down to its bitter end. This means that you don't end the scene in your soul writing script at the point where you experienced the agony, but carry on, if necessary, to the experience of not being able to talk to anyone about the pain (perhaps even to today) and how you endured this until you had to fall asleep, being obliged to function the following day.

10. Healing in the form of re-writing always first begins once you have the pain image in a scene on paper or in your computer. To this end you look for what you feel to be the peak of your suffering. Sometimes hushing it up is worse than the violence that one experienced. Take the point at which you sense that, if you don't change course and right now in the very next second begin to fight back, you'll never be free of it and you know how it will end – that's your project for today.

11. After this line in which the peak of your suffering is reached, you draw the proverbial red line. For this, you write at the end of your previous text that is where the re-writing begins.

a) The turnaround from the pain image to re-writing happens at exactly the moment in your narrative in which your pain is greatest. This makes it clear that all the lines thereafter, to the end of your story, no longer have any significance. However, you don't delete them; you want to remain aware that the agony you suffered is no longer to be swallowed to ultimately make you ill. Instead, here after the red line is where your new reality begins, the reality that will finally make you healthy and happy.

b) This new reality is not true in a rational sense, but it has an effect and that's the key. With the re-writing you produce new cell information or a new morphogenetic field. Both are highly effective and can immediately lead to a better constitution.

12. This is the reason you should not let too much time pass between writing the pain image and starting your re-writing. It is clear that the pain image, as the name implies, does not create good feelings. You might even experience a change for the worse, because you are now finally aware of what you have really suffered. This is why it is very important to begin immediately with the transformation of your suffering.

13. Only in the rarest of cases is a re-writing finished right away because the project (the symptom) has disappeared or the relationship has been harmonized Every re-writing has to be reworked a second or third or even a ninth time – after all we don't want half-hearted happiness, we want happiness in full. You can receive impetus for this in the shop or on the portal at clemenskuby.com if you find you aren't progressing, or you can begin anew with the drafting of your project. It is important for you to have a stable identity as a spirit-soul entity and to work with the KUBYmethod until you have achieved palpable success.

Divide your page into 4 columns using the table mode. 1st column (No.) ca. 3/8 in./1 cm: consecutive numbering of the lines in the table. 2nd column (Person) 1 in./3 cm: abbreviation for the person involved. 3rd column (Text) ca. 2 ¾ in./ 7 cm: the plot and the literal wording of the acting protagonists, written in the present tense. 4th column (Comments) 2 in./ 5 cm: left blank for improvements and comments.

1st Col.	**2nd Col.**	**3rd Col.**	**4th Col.**
No.	Person	Text	Comments
1	NN	Soul text in direct speech	....
2	NN	Soul text in the present tense	....

A. You begin a new line with every **change of the protagonist**.

B. The 3rd column in every line contains either what the protagonist (whose name is in the 2nd column) says, word for word in his or her own authentic speech; if necessary this can be in a foreign language or dialect.

C. Or you write in the 3rd column what the protagonist is doing at the moment if he or she is not saying anything.

D. If the protagonist is neither saying nor doing anything, you can write in the 3rd column: *He thinks: ....* Please do not lapse into explanations; instead, simply write briefly that NN, for instance, thinks: *I'd better not say anything now,* or *I'd like to scream but I can't,* etc.

E. Never speak of yourself in the third person. This is why the 2nd column never has your name in it, but "Me".

F. Because of the continuous numbering of your soul writing in the 1st column, please do not leave any blank lines in your text! And – this is IMPORTANT – never write more than 1,000 characters in one line. It is better to insert a line break more often than not often enough.

I hope that your soul writing goes smoothly; without these rules it cannot be a success.

All the best
Clemens Kuby

About the author

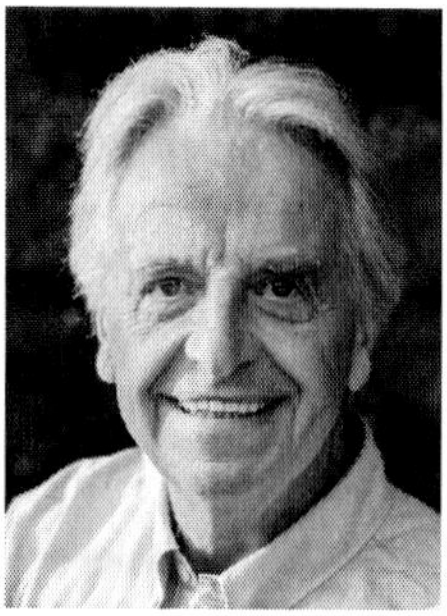

Clemens Kuby, born in 1947, award-winning documentary filmmaker (e.g. *Living Buddha*) and bestseller author, was paralysed and healed himself mentally. After this he learnt about the work of shamans and healers in 14 countries all over the world and documented them in his fascinating cult film and the bestseller of the same name, "*En route to the next dimension.*" In search for explanations for his so-called "miracle" or "spontaneous healing", as medicine calls it, he encountered serious findings in modern brain research and quantum physics, through which hitherto inexplicable healing phenomena can be understood.

With this knowledge and his own decades of experience with self-healing, Clemens Kuby developed *KUBYmethod* that can be applied to all people. For his method, Kuby reverts to his profound knowledge of film-making, which teaches him that reality does not have to be true, rather, reality is what has an effect – even if it is "only" imagined.

Many people have cured themselves with Clemens Kuby's books and films. If you would like to receive personal guidance from him, you can attend his lectures, workshops, and seminars, or arrange a online – session with him or with experts trained by him on the *KUBYmethod.*

Works by Clemens Kuby

On his most recent book: *Practised reincarnation – My incredible experiences*, Clemens Kuby has worked for 30 years. With the example of Jamgon Kontrul who had died in a car crash in 1992 and was reborn several years later, Kuby gives profound insights of how reincarnation works. He also shows us how to become aware of our former lives and how to plan our next life.

The bestseller *En route to the next Dimension* as a hardcover and paperback. Clemens Kuby's journey to healers and shamans. An overwhelming book.

The cult film *En route to the next Dimension* on DVD, 90 Min. This is *the* film about spiritual healing. You see what you have always suspected but never dared to believe.

The soundtrack for *Healing – the miracle inside you* on CD is healing music that impacts you by Büdi Siebert and friends from various cultures.

DVD: *Todas – on the edge of paradise.* A primordial tribe in South India who live the same way as they did thousands of years ago which Clemens Kuby visited several times over four years. They do not work and are without fear – fascinating!

DVD: *The Old Ladakh,* Buddhist Trilogy Part I. Tibetan culture as it once existed. A cult film, awarded with the German Film prize.

DVD: *Tibet – The Survival of the Spirit*, Buddhist Trilogy Part II. How the Tibetans can maintain their peaceful character despite Chinese occupation and brutality.

DVD: *Living Buddha*, Buddhist Trilogy Part III. A unique, monumental epic about a person in two lives, the 16th & 17th Gyalwa Karmapa.

DVD: *Making Of Living Buddha* + bonus material. This film is like a thriller in the way Kuby dealt with the greatest resistances while filming *Living Buddha* over seven years.

Contact

www.clemenskuby.com
For further information around the KUBYmethod:
help@kubymethod.com

For further information around our books & movies:
medienshop@clemenskuby.com

Made in United States
North Haven, CT
10 November 2026

22079722R00083